ANTI INFLAMMATORY DIET

Heal Your Body, Eat Healthy, and Reduce Inflammation

Contents

This document is geared towards providing exact and reliable information with regards to the topic and issue covered. The publication is sold with the idea that the publisher is not required to render accounting, officially permitted, or otherwise, qualified services. If advice is necessary, legal or professional, a practiced individual in the profession should be ordered.

A Declaration of Principles was accepted and approved equally by a Committee of the American Bar Association and a Committee of Publishers and Associations.

It is illegal to reproduce, duplicate, or transmit any part of this document in either electronic means or in printed format. Recording of this publication is strictly prohibited and any storage of this document is not allowed unless with written permission from the publisher.

The information provided herein is stated to be truthful and consistent, in that any liability, in terms of inattention or otherwise, by any usage or abuse of any policies, processes, or directions contained within, is the solitary and utter responsibility of the recipient reader. Under no circumstances will any legal responsibility or blame be held against the publisher for any reparation, damages, or monetary loss due to the information herein, either directly or indirectly.

Respective authors own all copyrights not held by the publisher.

The information herein is offered solely for informational purposes only, and is universal as so. The presentation of the information is not guaranteed.

The trademarks used are without any consent, and the publication of the trademark is without permission or backing by the trademark owner. All trademarks and brands within this book are for clarifying purposes only and are owned by the owners themselves, who are not affiliated with this document.

Disclaimer

All erudition contained in this book is given for informational and educational purposes only. The author is not in any way accountable for any results or outcomes that emanate from using this material. Constructive attempts have been made to provide information that is both accurate and effective, but the author is not bound for the accuracy or use/misuse of this information.

Foreword

First, I would like to thank you for taking the first step of trusting me and deciding to purchase/read this life-transforming eBook. Thank you for spending your time and resources on this material.

I can assure you of exact results, if you will diligently follow the exact blueprint, that I lay bare in the information manual you are currently reading. It has transformed lives, and I strongly believe it will equally transform your own life too.

All the information presented in this Do It Yourself piece is easy to digest and practice.

Book Description

Most individuals are conscious of mechanical causes of back pain like ligament sprains, muscle and strains, slipped disks, etc. Fewer individuals are conscious of inflammatory back pain, and also the simple fact that our diets may result in systemic inflammation, which contributes to pain through your body. It is essential to be educated concerning all manners of diet that may promote inflammation.

There is no doubt that people do not make good food options as a nation, according to the ever-increasing proportions of lifestyle and obesity disorders. The conventional American diet today depends mostly on "comfort foods" where generally 60 percent of those calories include oils, sugar and wheat. When these foods taste great, they have a high number of acids. Why should you take care of arachidonic acid?

Our body converts DHA to a chemical named Resolvin D2 that's a powerful anti-aging agent. It works by preventing the creation of pro-inflammatory eicosanoids that decrease the redness considerably and offer immediate relief from various ailments such as arthritis.

If you would like to earn this valuable fatty acid as part of your everyday diet, one great and effective manner is to incorporate superior fish oil supplements into your regimen. Be certain that you pick a product using more DHA material than EPA. This not only aids in ensuring that the anti-inflammatory properties in DHA, but also ensures a considerable supply of DHA and EPA into your system. This is a result of our body's capability to convert DHA to EPA according to its necessity.

In this book, you'll learn about:

- Anti-Inflammatory diet

- Food high in omega-6: omega-3 ratio

- Benefits of omega-3

- Healthier, stronger bones

- Improved mood regulation

- Reduced risk of Parkinson's

- Reduced risk of death from all causes

- Anti-Inflammatory foods and many more

Are you ready to explore the powerful DIY guide to heal your body, eat healthy, and reduce inflammation? Press the "BUY NOW" button and get started right away!

INTRODUCTION

Anti-inflammation is the property of a substance or treatment that diminishes irritation or swelling. Anti-inflammatory medications make up about portion of analgesics, curing of pains by diminishing inflammatory rather than narcotics, which influence the focal sensory system to square agony motioning to the cerebrum. The anti-inflammatory diet is an eating plan intended to counteract or diminish poor quality and ceaseless irritation, a key hazard factor in a large group of medical issues and a few noteworthy diseases. The run of the mill calming diet accentuates natural products, vegetables, lean protein, nuts, seeds and solid fats.

There is nobody's anti-inflammatory diet, rather, there are diets planned around nourishments that are accepted to diminish irritation and disregard sustenance that bother the incendiary procedures. Numerous anti-inflammatory diets are based around entire grains, vegetables, nuts, seeds, new vegetables and natural products, wild fish and fish, grass-encouraged slender turkey and chicken, which are thought to help in the bodies mending of aggravation. They prohibit nourishments that are thought to trigger aggravation, for example, refined grains, wheat, corn, full-fat dairy, red meat, caffeine , liquor, peanuts, sugar, immersed and trans-soaked fats.

The impacts of the anti-inflammatory diet are subtle. There is progressive research that exhibits an advantage in the decrease of perpetual ailments, for example, cardiovascular ailment, neurodegenerative sicknesses, and malignant growths when following a dietary example related with the calming diet. Nonetheless, the advantages go past sickness aversion. Studies have demonstrated enlightening side effects related with ceaseless infections. Also, an individual may diminish or cease their dose of drugs endorsed to control side effects identified with provocative conditions, and lessen the side influences related with calming specialists.

It has likewise been recorded that individuals who pursued the calming diet expressed they had encountered loss of weight, a rise of vitality, and revealed better mental and passionate wellbeing.

The normal establishment of anti-inflammatory diets is the conviction that low evaluations of irritation are the forerunner as well as antagonizes numerous unending ailments. When evacuated, the body can start mending itself. The philosophical beginning of anti-inflammatory diets goes back to the first healers from the beginning of time who have worked with nourishments, herbs, teas and other characteristic solutions, for helping the body's very own mending vitality.

Endless ailment — an ailment that endures over an extensive stretch of time and sometimes causes a long haul change in the body.

C-receptive protein (CRP) — a marker of irritation flowing in the blood that has been proposed as a technique to recognize people in danger of these sicknesses.

Flavonoid — alludes to mixes found in natural products, vegetables, and certain refreshments that have differing biochemical and cancer prevention agents.

Inflammation

Different nourishments are utilized in an unexpected way, some advancing inflammation while others diminish it. The motivation behind the calming diet is to advance ideal wellbeing and mending by picking nourishments that lessen irritation. In the event that one can effectively control extreme irritation through normal methods (for example, a eating regimen), it lessens one's reliance on calming prescriptions that have undesirable and unfortunate symptoms that don't take care of the fundamental issue. While anti-inflammatory drugs, (for example, NSAIDs) are a convenient solution to ease manifestations, they debilitate the invulnerable framework by harming the gastrointestinal tract,.

Inflammation is a restricted response of tissue to damage, regardless of whether it was brought about by microscopic organisms or viral disease, injury, synthetics, heat or other marvels that cause disturbance. The 'disturbance' makes the tissues inside the body discharge numerous substances. This perplexing reaction is called aggravation.

Inflammation is portrayed by such manifestations that incorporate:

(1) Vasodilatation of the close veins which brings about abundance to the local blood stream

(2) Increases in the penetrability of the vessels with spillage of enormous amounts of liquid into the interstitial spaces

(3) Coagulation of the fluid in the interstitial spaces due to the abundant measures of fibrinogen and different proteins spilling from the vessels

(4) Relocation of granulocytes and monocytes into the tissue in enormous quantities

(5) Swelling of the tissue cells

The regular substances discharged from the tissues that outcome in inflammation are histamine, bradykinin, serotonin, prostaglandins, and numerous hormonal substances that are considered as lymphokines, which are discharged by sharpened T-cells and different responses inside the body. A considerable amount of these substances actuate the macrophage framework, which are conveyed to discard the harmed tissue, yet additionally further harm the living tissue and cells.

CHAPTER ONE

What Does An Anti-Inflammatory Diet Do?

An anti-inflammatory diet comprises of nourishments that lessen inflammatory reactions. This eating regimen includes supplanting sugary, refined nourishments with entire, supplement rich sustenance. Anti-inflammatory diet contains expanded measures of cancer prevention agents, which are responsive particles in nourishment that diminish the quantity of free radicals. They are atoms in the body that may harm cells and are incremental to the danger of specific infections.

Numerous famous weight control plans now pursue calming standards. For instance, the Mediterranean eating routine contains fish, entire grains, and fats that are useful for the heart. Research has demonstrated that this eating regimen can decrease the impacts of aggravation on the cardiovascular framework.

The body's resistant framework is intended to fend off dangers, similar to disease causing germs, through a procedure called irritation. Be that as it may, a relentless condition of irritation can prompt everything from diabetes to immune system infections to coronary illness to malignancy. Huge numbers of these wellbeing dangers do not originate from remote intruders like terrifying microscopic organisms, yet from some ordinary sustenance you are most likely eating. When expelling irritation, you are inciting sustenance from your eating regimen, or if nothing else restricting them, it can enable you to make a superior showing of ensuring your prosperity.

For a considerable lot of the most widely recognized unending illnesses prodded by inflammation, the beginning stage is heftiness. What's more, corpulence is regularly the consequence of indulging sustenance that encourages inflammation. Most—however not all—of the nourishments that reason aggravation convey negligible sustenance. Handled sustenance made with refined white flour and white sugar are top of the guilty parties. These incorporate bundled white breads and rolls, heated merchandise and treats. Soft drinks and other sugar-improved beverages are in a similar classification. Fats, for example, margarine, also advance inflammation, and so do prepared red meats, hotdogs, sausage, salami and other store meats. Indeed, even lean red meat ought to be constrained to on more than one occasion per week.

Inflammation

Inflammation is a characteristic procedure with the natural reason to start mending by expanding dissemination. It is a mind boggling procedure that includes both the safe framework and vascular framework and the transaction of different substances. Expanded course brings white platelets and sustenance to the site of damage or contamination with the goal that attacking pathogens are murdered and harm might be fixed. Trademark indications of irritation incorporate torment (dolor), heat (calor), swelling (tumor) and redness (rubor).

In wide terms, inflammation is the body's safe framework's reaction to a stimulus. This can be because of normal wounds, for example, consuming your finger, or tumbling off of a bike, after which you feel the influenced zone become red, warm, and puffy. This is a confined reaction to damage, described by 'expanded blood stream, hair-like enlargement, leucocyte invasion, and generation of synthetic mediators.' In short, a fiery reaction implies the natural (vague) safe framework is 'battling against something that may end up being unsafe.'

Notably, while inflammation is frequently thrown in a negative light, it is really basic in limiting quantities for insusceptible observation and host defense. In evident of the 'Goldilocks' structure, excessively little and a lot of inflammation both posture issues; truth be told, most unending sicknesses are believed to be established in second rate irritation that perseveres after some time. This irritation may go unnoticed by the host (you!) until clear pathologies emerge, which incorporate, and are not restricted to, diabetes, cardiovascular sickness, nonalcoholic greasy liver infection, weight, immune system issues, incendiary entrails illness, and even clinical misery. This idea is called 'The aggravation hypothesis of ailment,' which irritation is the regular hidden factor among the main sources of death.

There are atoms in the body called prostaglandins which assume a significant job in irritation. It has been discovered that of the three fundamental kinds of prostaglandins, two of them (PG-E1 and PG-E3) have a mitigating impact, while the third sort (PG-E2) really advances aggravation. At the point when there is a lopsidedness in the body between these prostaglandins, aggravation can result. Prostaglandins are made in the body from fundamental unsaturated fats. You can help your body in making calming prostaglandins by eating vegetables, nuts, grains and seeds, for example, sesame and sunflower seeds. Then again, foods that reason a spike in insulin levels, for example, sugary nourishments, or nourishments with a high glycemic burden advance generation of PG-E2 and increment aggravation, can affect the body too.

An ordinary mitigating diet centers around battling irritation through the utilization of foods that lower insulin levels. To effectively lessen irritation, you ought to eat nourishments that have a low glycemic load, for example, entire grains, vegetables and lentils, and expend sound fats, for example, nuts, seeds, fish, additional virgin olive oil and fish. Flavors such as turmeric, ginger, and hot peppers, additionally decrease irritation. Simultaneously, you need to diminish utilization of foods that are genius incendiary, like red meat, egg yolks and shellfish. Sugar is a key offender in aggravation, and you should curtail sugary nourishments. Irritation can be decreased by taking enhancements, for example, fish oils which are high in omega-3 and unsaturated fats.

At the point when inflammation goes awry:

While some inflammation is valuable and fitting for recuperating, endless or intemperate inflammation, filling no need produces harm. Interminable inflammation has a terrible notoriety since it is involved in different ailment procedures including (however not restricted to):

- Autoimmune sicknesses

- Joint pain

- Diabetes

- Alzheimer's sickness

- Atherosclerosis (solidifying of supply routes that prompts heart assault and stroke)

- ADD and ADHD

- Hypersensitivities and asthma

- Cancer

- Inflammation gut sickness

Delicate tissue swelling and people engaged with aggravation can likewise disturb nerve endings, adding to torment.

What makes up an anti-inflammatory diet?

Drawn-out second rate inflammation is related with extreme oxidative pressure and changed glucose and lipid digestion in our (fat) cells, muscle and liver. Therefore, investigation recommends that specific dietary parts can tweak these key incendiary pathways and clinical pathologies. It is clarified that anti-inflammatory diet is the comprehension of how individual supplements can influence the equivalent atomic targets by pharmacological medications.

Convincing research from an enormous scale, longitudinal observational examinations, including the Women's Health Initiative Observational Study and Multi-Ethnic Study of Atherosclerosis (MESA) study, suggest that a diet with fitting calories that is low in refined starches, high in dissolvable fiber, high in mono unsaturated fats, a higher omega-3 to omega-6 proportion, and high in polyphenols, all have calming consequences for the body. A Mediterranean eating regimen design that joins olive oil, fish, humble lean meat utilization, and rich products of the soil, vegetables, and entire grains, indicates increasingly mitigating impacts when contrasted with an ordinary American dietary example. Other observational and interventional studies have additionally proposed that dietary examples joining green and dark tea, pecans, ground flaxseed and garlic are likewise connected with decreased aggravation.

Correspondence between the fundamental insusceptible framework and the focal sensory system (CNS) is a basic, however regularly neglected segment of the fiery reaction to tissue damage, illness or infection.

Social investigations have demonstrated that delayed mental pressure can actuate the similar genius fiery pathways we've been talking about from the beginning. While unending mental pressure can advance over-articulation of expert fiery arbiters, it can likewise advance indulging unhealthful sustenance without craving. Repetitive stress-eating, calorie-thick, supplements of poor sustenance not only worsens the mental pain and makes an endless loop of pressure eating, it also advances adiposity, which we've portrayed is a genius fiery state.

In all honesty, inflammation begins as something to be thankful for. It happens when your invulnerable framework conveys white platelets and "warrior" mixes like eicosanoids to assault attacking infections, microorganisms or poisons. An exemplary case of absolutely ordinary inflammation: torment, warmth, redness and swelling around an injury or damage (think about a delicate sprained lower leg).

There's a different reaction called 'goals' that takes the pooches of war back to their sleeping quarters and recuperates your tissues. The main period of inflammation causes cell decimation, and the subsequent stage, goals, starts cell revival. For whatever length of time that those stages are adjusted, you remain well.

However, for increasingly more of us, the parity never occurs. That is on the grounds that sugar, refined grains, and soaked fat can likewise trigger an inflammatory immune reaction, and the commonplace Western eating routine is pressed with them, which means we're inflaming our bodies again and again, every time we eat. In the meantime, think about what the normal American gets excessively little of: leafy foods, dull veggies, which are stuffed with cell reinforcements that help chill things off and diminish the force of the underlying inflammatory reaction, and greasy fish, an incredible wellspring of omega-3 unsaturated fats, which can help move your body into the goals stage.

Air contamination and natural poisons trigger your inflammatory immune responses along these lines, yet the greater part of the ceaseless, additional irritation in our bodies is diet-related. Endless inflammation can prompt coronary illness. In the mind, it is connected to tension and gloom. In your joints, it causes swelling and torment. In the gut, inflammation loses the equalization of supportive microscopic organisms and makes direct harm when covering the digestion tracts.

Irritation and diet

You most likely have known about anti-inflammatory drugs. In any case, did you realize that there is a relationship that exists among irritation and diet? Undoubtedly, there is such an unbelievable marvel as a calming diet, which comprises of nourishments that counteract the beginning of inflammation.

Inflammation is essentially a restricted response of the cells and tissues in light of bothering, contamination or damage. It is portrayed by agony, red shading and swelling, with genuine conditions joined by loss of development or even work. Basic inflammation conditions we know incorporate joint inflammation and gout, however constant maladies, for example, coronary illness and stroke, can be ascribed to some type of inflammation.

Ongoing exploration about today connects inflammation to a wide scope of ceaseless ailments. Heart sicknesses, sorrow, diabetes, and feed fever appear to be different as far as side effects, however they all make inflammation. Thus, fostering a strategic distance from ceaseless infections connected to irritation, it is then critical to counteract and switch harm that this foundational aggravation can cause. What's more, indeed, you are correct; this should be possible through a solid, adjusted, mitigating diet.

The meals we eat can influence inflammation in an unusually intricate way. The best counsel to pursue this is to keep away from 'star incendiary foods' or nourishments that expand inflammation, and take in a greater amount of mitigating sustenance sources. This implies taking less of soaked fats found in meats, eggs, and dairy items which are wealthy in inflammation and advance arachidonic corrosive, while taking more or low-fat milk, lean meat, fish and vegetables. It is essential to abstain from taking in an excessive amount of sugar as it isn't just identified with inflammation, it also is affected by heftiness and numerous other unending ailments.

The advantages of keeping up a sound eating regimen, free of expert provocative mixes, don't just liberate you from the danger of creating irritation and conditions that go with it, but also gives you long haul benefits. In the end, you will acknowledge how a decent calming eating regimen can make your skin look more youthful, expel the hypersensitivity side effects, make your joints feel much improved, and give you a general solid inclination.

Omega-3, unsaturated fats in fish oil, are one of the most significant viewpoints in a sound, anti-inflammatory diet. These basic unsaturated fats are extremely intense anti-inflammatory specialists that can shield and ease you from all types of inflammation. You can get your daily portion of omega-3 fish oils through admission of satisfactory measures of fish, or by taking an ordinary portion of fish oil supplements. Make a point to counsel with your nutritionist or specialist in regards to a suitable dose.

Beside the solid connection among irritation and diet, look into concentrates that additionally propose the significance of driving the way towards life's propensities. For example, practicing normally, keeping up a perfect weight, limiting pressure, and evasion of smoking and liquor.

Chronic inflammation and diet

Late examinations have demonstrated that ceaseless irritation could, to a limited extent, be in charge of the advancement of ailments like malignant growth, alzheimer's infection, and rheumatoid joint inflammation.

What causes unending inflammation? Grouped factors are evidently at fault. For instance, poisons, stress, latency, less than stellar eating routines, and hereditary qualities are a portion of the presumed offenders.

In what capacity can endless inflammation be tended to? Here are some dietary approaches to lessen the hazard.

• **Food decisions.** What we put in our bodies assumes a noteworthy job in our prosperity. Individuals who routinely devour inexpensive food, handled meats, greasy tidbits, and oily suppers, don't charge so well on the wellbeing scale than people who eat carefully. Actually, these individuals are leaving themselves open to an expanded danger of corpulence, elevated cholesterol, diabetes and other undesirable conditions. To put it plainly, sustenance matters! Which choices will be ideal? Matured soy, verdant vegetables, grouped mushrooms, new natural products, extra-virgin olive oil, cold-water fish, green and dark tea, nuts and red wine (with some restraint) are great decisions. Simultaneously, it is imperative to purchase natural products. As we are probably aware, natural yields are those that have not been splashed with pesticides.

• **Vitamins and supplements.** Normally, the ideal path for getting basic nutrients, minerals and supplements in the body is by eating entire foods: crisp vegetables and natural products are particularly great decisions. In any case, customary access to crisp sustenance isn't constantly feasible for certain individuals. Along these lines, fantastic enhancements might be required. Which types are best in battling irritation? Ones that contain nutrients C, D, and E, folic corrosive, selenium, carotenoids, fish oil, coQ10, turmeric or curcumin, garlic and ginger. NOTE: Always check with your PCP before taking enhancements. Particular sorts may meddle with prescriptions or intensify the impacts of specific medications (like blood thinners).

• **Fiber.** Fiber merits a class all on its own, and its advantages are stunning. Standard admission of this miracle has been thought to diminish conditions like coronary illness, elevated cholesterol and certain malignancies. Which sort of fiber is best in battling aggravation? The dissolvable assortment like those found in beans, oat grain, lentils, apples, nuts, seeds and strawberries. Insoluble sorts like those found in entire grains and wheat grain additionally fill a need since they will, in general, get things going along in our stomach related tract. Taking in the middle of 25 to 35 grams of fiber for every day, with roughly 2/3's originating from the dissolvable grouping, is believed to be certain. Strikingly, while different starches similar to white flour and sugar, ought to be disregarded, however much could be expected. Solvent fiber carbs are unquestionably not miscreants.

There are different approaches to limit inflammation in spite of nourishment. Exercise, yoga and hurling the cigarettes (and when you smoke), help strengthen a calming diet.

Some ideas on how an anti-inflammatory diet works

There is anything but a formal eating regimen plan that frameworks precisely what to eat, its amount and when. Or maybe, the mitigating diet is tied in with filling your suppers with nourishment that have been appeared to battle aggravation and — similarly as significant — removing nourishments that have been appeared to add to it.

When thinking about the mitigating diet as a way of life as opposed to an eating routine: "A calming diet is an eating plan that attempts to diminish or limit poor quality aggravation inside our bodies."

In a perfect world, you would eat seven to nine servings of leafy foods every day, limit your admission of red meat and dairy, pick complex sugars over straightforward ones and swear off handled sustenance.

You'll need to pick nourishments that are wealthy in omega-3 unsaturated fats — including anchovies, salmon, halibut, and mussels — as opposed to omega-6 unsaturated fats, which are found in corn oil, vegetable oil, mayonnaise, plate of mixed greens dressings and many prepared meals.

Eating along these lines is a smart thought for everybody on the grounds that huge numbers of the nourishments, with the possibility to prompt irritation, aren't sound at any rate. Everybody can profit by constraining or disposing of sugar, and exceptionally handled foods, and instead add unsaturated fats, organic products, vegetables, nuts, seeds, and slender proteins to their diet.

The anti-inflammatory diet could be particularly useful for somebody who is managing interminable irritation because of a wellbeing condition. Competitors and individuals who exercise at a high power, and are hoping to decrease their standard irritation, could also think that it is valuable.

Step by step instructions to recognize anti-inflammatory diet

In any case, the arrangement with the most research-sponsored anti-inflamatory cred is the customary Mediterranean eating regimen, underscoring natural products, vegetables, entire grains, vegetables, fish and olive oil. A few extremely enormous investigations—including the renowned Nurses' Health Study—have discovered that individuals who pursue a Mediterranean example of eating have lower levels of the incendiary markers C-responsive protein and interleukin-6 in their blood contrasting to the individuals who don't. This might be one reason the Mediterranean eating routine is connected to such a large number of medical advantages, from holding weight down to cutting heart and stroke chance.

The objectives of an AI plan are basic: cut route back on foods that trigger an incendiary reaction and eat a greater amount of the nourishments that mend harm. While there are a few varieties in what's permitted and what isn't, most AI plans share an accentuation on eating entire, insignificantly prepared nourishments, non-dull vegetables, monounsaturated fats like olive oil and avocado, beautiful berries and other organic product, and loads of omega-3s from greasy fish (or enhancements) and staying away from included sugar and refined grains.

All things considered, your plate may appear to be somewhat unique from your companion's or coworker's, and that is the manner in which it ought to be. Meal sensitivities assume a job, as well:

people respond to nourishments in an unexpected way, and in the event that somebody has an affectability to a specific nourishment, it will prompt cytokine creation and an expansion in other incendiary synthetic concoctions.

Who should eat the anti-inflammatory diet?

Did you know that inflammation has been recognized as the basis for most chronic diseases such as arthritis, obesity, diabetes, obesity, heart disease and even cancer? That's appropriate. These food choices are set to perform a host of processes within your body which produce inflammation by a number of sources. Additionally, many of us are genetically programmed to produce excessive redness when subjected to ordinary irritant sources like smoke, chemicals and poor nutritional choices.

How exactly do poor food choices create inflammation? Highly processed and packaged products like fast foods are some of the worst offenders. They're also a number of the food options that are most broadly offered. Designed for ease, these meals are filled with trans-fat to extend their shelf life in addition to change their taste and feel. A trans-fat is made out of a standard, saturated fat, yet another less than healthful fat. This saturated fat is 'transformed' to a trans-fat with a procedure known as trans-hydrogenation. This transformed fat, when incorporated into your body, makes a cascade of substances called cytokines.

Foods that contains refined sugars are also inflammatory. Cakes, biscuits and doughnuts are examples of foods that are rapidly digested by the human body, releasing large amounts of glucose. This sugar is quickly absorbed by your body, causing a high blood glucose level. Your body consequently produces a surge of insulin to help normalize your blood sugar levels. This surge of insulin, combined with higher blood glucose levels, causes the human body to release cytokines, inflammatory compounds as well. Guess what? Fat tissue becomes more active and starts to release the identical inflammatory molecules, cytokines, too.

Processed grains stripped of fiber and other vital nutrients also create inflammation. A whole grain is a molecule composed of considerable amounts of sugar linked together and encapsulated using a fiber coat. This fiber coating makes the digestion and release of sugar a slow and continuous procedure. If the outer fiber coating has been stripped off to create a smooth and creamy texture, sugar molecules are easily available for quick digestion and absorption in your body. This rapid surge of sugar into your system is the cause for the inflammatory cascade.

Particular grains have the ability to produce inflammation in certain people. Wheat, barley, oats and rye are all grains that contain significant quantities of a protein substance called gluten free. Gluten makes foods, like bread, crispy on the outside and tender on the inside. Yet this identical gluten is extremely inflammatory in individuals genetically challenged in digesting gluten free. Symptoms can be as intense as pain, bloating, diarrhea and malnutrition, or as moderate as nausea or deficiency of energy. Eliminating these particular grains from your diet is often the key to controlling this sort of inflammation.

Generally, an anti-inflammatory diet is composed of fresh whole foods, which do not include causes for inflammation, and are packed with molecules which neutralize inflammation in the human system.

Phytonutrients are found in most fruits and vegetables, and are responsible for their vivid look. These massive molecules include antioxidants as well as anti-inflammatory properties. This implies that they neutralize the oxidative stress your body generates daily, leading to inflammation. Healthy fats found in cold water, oily fish, flax seed and nuts can also diminish the quantity of inflammation produced by the human body as well. Cooking oils such as olive oil and canola oil also help your body combat and neutralize inflammation. These antioxidants also repel oxidative stress and soften the formation of melancholy.

Eliminating foods that are fast in addition to packed foods is the initial step of this anti-inflammatory diet. Eliminating foods with processed sugars and processed carbs is the next step. Eating generous daily quantities of fruit and vegetables as well as moderate amounts of whole grains and lean protein, in addition to healthful fats found in fish, seeds and nuts, is the basis of the anti-inflammatory diet. Then for select people, reducing or eliminating grains, particularly gluten-containing grains, would be the final step.

So who must eat an anti-inflammatory diet? Or what advantages in allergic disorders (eczema, asthma) will people gain in the anti-inflammatory diet? Many people with chronic pain (headaches, back pain, neck pain, knee pain, joint pains, and nerve pains, muscle pains) have components of inflammation involved in their pain, will benefit from this too. Irritable bowel syndrome, along with common digestive disorders like acid reflux, improve with the anti-inflammatory diet. In the end, anyone interested in preventing those degenerative ailments and attaining optimal health will gain improvement. In fact, the science confirms that eating to reduce inflammation not merely prevents illness and keeps health, but it also keeps us looking and feeling younger.

What the research says

There's a lot of research demonstrating the negative impacts of inflammation. It's related with medical problems from diabetes and Alzheimer's to disease and weight.

A few different investigations have taken a look at the impact of a daily eating routine wealthy in anti-inflammatory nourishments. For example, picking calming nourishments may help individuals with rheumatoid joint pain (RA). Following an eating routine like this won't really fix you, yet it might help decrease the malady's effect, defer movement, diminish how much drug is required and lessen joint harm.

Different investigations have discovered anti-inflammatory nourishments can:

• Help competitors recuperate

• Manage agony related with maturing

• Protect the heart

• Improve personal satisfaction for individuals with numerous sclerosis

A food list of what to eat on an anti-inflammatory diet

Following anti-inflammatory diet means stacking up on nourishments which examinations have indicated can help lower irritation, and that diminishing your admission of meals can have a contrary impact. The best thing about the eating regimen is there are a lot of sustenance alternatives and bunches of squirm room so you can pick the nourishments you like best.

In the event that you need more structure, consider embracing the Mediterranean eating regimen. There's a great deal of cover with the calming diet in light of the fact that both underscore eating organic products, vegetables and entire grains.

Nourishments to eat

• Fresh organic product, including grapefruit, grapes, blueberries, bananas, apples, mangos, peaches, tomatoes, and pomegranates

• Dried organic product, including plums

• Vegetables, particularly broccoli, brussels sprouts, cauliflower, and bok choy

• Plant-based proteins, for example, chickpeas, seitan and lentils

• Fatty fish, for example, salmon, sardines, tuna fish, herring, lake trout and mackerel

• Whole grains, including oats, dark colored rice, grain and entire wheat loaf

• Leafy greens, including spinach, romaine lettuce and kale

• Ginger

• Nuts, including pecans and almonds

• Seeds, for example, chia seeds and flaxseed

• Foods loaded up with omega-3 unsaturated fats, for example, avocado and olive oil

• Coffee

• Green tea

• Dark chocolate (with some restraint)

• Red wine (with some restraint)

What conditions can a mitigating diet help with?

Specialists, dietitians and naturopaths prescribe calming eats less carbs as an integral treatment for some conditions that are intensified by unending aggravation.

A mitigating diet can support numerous conditions, including:

• Rheumatoid joint pain

• Psoriasis

• Asthma

• Eosinophilic esophagitis

• Crohn's sickness

• Colitis

• Inflammatory inside illness

• Diabetes

• Obesity

• Metabolic disorder

• Heart sickness

- Lupus

- Hashimoto's sickness

Also, eating a mitigating diet can help diminish the danger of specific malignant growths, including colorectal disease.

Health Benefits of Following an Anti-Inflammatory Diet?

Following a calming diet has appeared to help individuals with:

- Autoimmune issue

- Heart malady

- Cancer, including bosom malignancy and colorectal disease

- Alzheimer's malady

- Diabetes

- Pulmonary malady

- Epilepsy

CHAPTER TWO

Nutritional Necessities

The significance of balanced diet in most inflammatory conditions

Let us quickly review the main causes of melancholy to be able to know the importance of a balanced diet plan. As we've already discussed a number of the most usual kinds of inflammation are: disease, allergies, environmental consequences, injury, psychological injury, nutrient deficiencies and excesses.

Infection: When an infection happens in the machine, it's because a fungus, bacterium, sediment, virus, or a different type of parasite assaulting the machine. The immune system prepares for conflict and responds with an inflammation that's particularly designed to attack the disease.

Allergy: Previously mentioned, an allergic reaction happens when the system responds to some material (possibly harmful or benign) which could potentially be a danger to your system. This might be anything from a particular foodto an insect bite. The body reacts with inflammation for a means to guard your system. Reactions may vary from moderate to intense.

It may happen when cells have been subjected to physical or chemical irritants. Many toxins (chlorine, pesticides, medications, asbestos, etc) could possibly result in harm to physical tissue. Continual exposure often leads to inflammation for a means to protect and cure the affected regions. Inflammation is an effective method for your human body to heal and repair cells in which were injured.

Psychological trauma: Anxiety and stress can have a negative influence on the body. Emotional distress has an immediate connection with an individual's physiology. As soon as a person undergoes psychological stress raised levels, cortisone and adrenaline are published and could lead to an imbalance and imbalance. Aging has a propensity to make the situation worse. The overload is usually more than the human body is well prepared to take care of. When a man is in great health, toxins are far more easily flushed out of the system.

Nutritional deficiency and nutritional excessive: Adrenal ailments, taxed immune system and inflammation are often connected to imbalances in nourishment. Nutritional deficiencies such as a lack of the correct fats, carbs, minerals and vitamins can leave the machine lacking in the nutrients required for tissue and cell restoration. Alternately, excessive quantities of specific foods may result in a nutrient imbalance, which could place unwanted pressure the bodily organs and tissues.

Factors come in to play: Psychological wellbeing, exercise, ecological conditions, lifestyle factors together with a genetic disposition and diet. As soon as we create a point of lessening our household's exposure to toxins, we become more mindful of how we handle our own body, and seeing what we consume can give ourselves a heightened capacity to take care of potentially threatening ailments.

Difference between true hunger and cravings

Hunger is a built in device that makes it possible for us to tune to our own body's unique nutritional demands. When someone encounters food cravings, normally there might be a nutrient deficiency. A craving for salty foods, as by way of instance, can signal a salt reduction. But several food cravings have a psychological component; frequently when individuals are dieting and trying to remove a specific kind, they may undergo cravings for the food.

Say, as an example, you have already been in the practice of eating a bag of fries while still sitting on the PC during the day. Should you opt to cut that action from our regular, you are very likely to experience a period in which you crave chips. A fantastic approach to decide on whether you're going through real thirst or a craving would be to envision replacing the chips with a different kind of food, say a apple. . .if the concept of this apple pleases the requirement, it is more than likely you're having is true thirst. If only chips will do. . .you're probably suffering from a food craving (Occasionally there's an underlying condition which may call for a health evaluation).

When someone eats for the ideal reasons they're usually eating when they're genuinely hungry and will stop eating if they're fulfilled, rather than too full. Ordinarily, a satisfying diet may consist of nutritious food whilst not filling out foods which appreciate capable. But when an individual becomes dominated by food cravings, then there's a propensity to add weight, overeat and endure nutritionally.

Understand how to keep an eye on your own food intake

The easiest way to remain in tune with our own body would be by keeping a food diary. A food diary permits you to keep tabs on our consumption habits. It's possible to record how you are feeling before ingestion, whilst eating, and also after ingestion. Keep tabs on how hungry you are at different phases every day.

By getting connected with patterns and triggers, you will quickly have the ability to comprehend and avoid giving into emotional cravings. If feelings get the best of you, you could have the ability to substitute that bag of fries using gluten free snacks (I've included a sample diary page in the conclusion of the segment).

Emotions and ingestion patterns are closely connected. Your diary will help make connections between feelings and eating customs. With practice, it is possible to substitute eating foods which cause inflammation, along with gluten free foods, which help promote optimum health. Gluten free recipes and meal programs contained in this publication will offer healthy choices. As you tune to your true nutrient needs, you're very likely to feel healthier whatsoever.

Another tip is to get a relative or friend to make the adjustments. In my situation, my spouse and I started following a gluten free app together. After the contents of the cabinets and fridge started to alter, we left each choice collectively. If one of us sensed that the need to get an unhealthy bite, another had been there to indicate the healthy choices.

Initially it had been rather slow moving, but as spouses, we turned into a united front and consequently simulated healthy changes and behaviors for our kids! Though my spouse and I maintain very hectic schedules, we store and cook at least one time each week. We utilize this time to search for specials and test new gluten free snacks.

Recognizing the root of inflammation and coeliac disease

Although it is good to know how food and allergies are linked to inflammation, it will help to comprehend the way digestion occurs in the digestive tract. Each time we eat, the food will be ground up from our teeth. Then it travels down the esophagus into your stomach and will be further divided, from antioxidants and enzymes, into a gentle paste-like material. The meals then travel to the tiny intestines in which the nutrients are consumed. The rest of the digested foods travels to the intestines and the most of the past remnants of water and salt are consumed before the waste is removed from the body. This procedure can occur between 24 and 72 hours based on the overall wellbeing of their intestines.

This description is very fundamental, and the full procedure is a lot more involved than what I have explained. The purpose is that if all is functioning in a wholesome fashion, proteins are divided up into single amino acids and fats are summoned in fatty acids, and carbohydrates have been divided into simple sugars. When all is in great working order, these nutrients are properly absorbed without inducing an allergic response. But when the cells lining the intestinal tract are more pliable, there might be a consequent imbalance along with a strong chance that the food cannot be properly digested.

Food allergies and coeliac disease

Since I've said, this explanation is simplified. On the other hand, the point I wish to stress is that there's an immediate connection between food allergies (especially in this instance to gluten) and several health ailments like arthritis, asthma, eczema, obesity and heart ailments. Since over 70 percent of the cells, which support the human immune system, are in the lining of the gastrointestinal tract, so it is not surprising that if food is not right for our wants, your body is going to be thrown right into a manner of attack. When many foods are healthful, foods, which you're allergic to, are reacted to such as toxins, the dangerous invaders. Blood flow increases along with the intestines becoming swollen.

Coeliac disease (or even Celiac disease) is among the conditions that could result in the body's inability to block the inflammation process from the gastrointestinal tract. The consequent fatigue and pain are symptoms of this small intestine's problem in consuming suitable nutrition. While this occurs, they respond to particular food particles as foreign materials. Among the most important causes of this illness would be gluten sensitivity or, to put it differently, gluten intolerance which could frequently be remedied using a gluten free diet.

CHAPTER THREE

Chronic Disease, Pain and Gluten

Heart disease and hypertension

I use the term disease widely to include different conditions like stroke, hypertension, heart attack, atherosclerosis, diabetes and higher blood pressure. When there are many risk factors related to cardiovascular disease, inflammation is also regarded among these. Damage to the adrenal tissues leads to microscopic tissue damage. As stated previously, low-grade inflammation, which happens over a time period, is known to raise the possibility of infection to the center. Whatever disturbs the equilibrium of this circulatory (heart) cells could possibly boost the possibility of cardiovascular disease.

Epithelial cells, which line blood vessels, restrain the circulation of hormones, nutrients, and also resistant facilitators that help regulate blood circulation, appropriate performance of the circulatory system and modulate blood pressure. The cells which help to support the immune system aid to safeguard the fragile tissues from strikes. Chronic inflammation is the most common crime to appropriate cardiovascular function.

Chronic pain and insomnia

Lots of types of persistent pain, such as fibromyalgia, may be the consequence of inflammation. Though fibromyalgia does not fall under the class of inflammatory disorder, among the indicators of this disease is inflammation. For individuals suffering from fibromyalgia, interrupted sleep patterns occur daily. We are aware that the immune system operates 24/7, cleansing our method and making fixes, particularly if we sleep. When sleep is upset, because it is for a lot of men and women who suffer with fibromyalgia, this cleansing/repair procedure isn't able to operate at the best level.

Why gluten free?

If this handicap of the cleansing/repair process happens, cells suffer from protracted inflammation due to the insufficient cleaning inside the system. Waste products start to accumulate. For a lot of men and women who suffer with this illness, serotonin levels change. This shift can negatively affect mood, sleep, and fresh tissue development, along with the metabolism of carbs essential for energy throughout the day. People with fibromyalgia have to have a healthier digestive tract.

A wholesome gluten free diet may offset this negative cycle and reduce the disagreeable gluten symptoms of this disease by reducing inflammation.

When the gastrointestinal system is working satisfactorily, inflammation is significantly decreased and dopamine secretions improve. This may elevate a individual's disposition and permit for quality of sleep. The positive consequence is the immune-system's capability to wash and repair the body through the night. The gluten free diet program is well known by several health professionals as an efficient means to help eliminate chronic pain and sleeplessness.

Gluten is a mix of plant fats found in lots of grains and other food items.

Gluten-free diets are made to contain all types of meals, which contain considerable quantities of gluten.

Gluten could be found in corn, and rice contain gluten free but in a form, which does not activate celiac disease, are believed to be gluten free.

While all meats include some kind of gluten free, gluten-free normally means foods that don't contain rye, barley, and wheat.

How is inflammation linked to allergy?

Generally, allergies result once the immune system (over) responds to foreign materials. A healthy immune system is about to guard the body in the intrusion of any undesirable agent in your system. After effective, the immune system shields our body against disease and infection.

But since the immune system isn't necessarily able to distinguish between good, impartial, and dangerous invaders, it is inclined to over-react. This hyperactive immunity may cause the human body to go to a tail-spin and respond to 'benign visitors' with protracted inflammation.

All these 'visitors' are called allergens. Resulting inflammation might happen abruptly or persist, resulting in moderate to severe allergic reactions.

What's a histamine?

When an individual has an illness, the body creates antibodies as a means to guard itself. Consequently, innumerable radicals attach to the face of the tissues inside physiological tissue.

There they wait to find the next attack via an allergen, which the body has recognized as a possible threat.

Assorted compounds in blood as it circulates throughout our body, leading to inflammation.

When another attack happens, the allergen is obligated by specific cells and a chemical is discharged. Histamine, among these specially designed compounds, results in the allergic reaction setup inside your own body. Histamine is associated with coughing, runny noses, itching and a number of the other distress related to allergic reactions.

Anti-allergy allergic reactions have two stages. There's an early stage, generated when the compounds are released, that may occur immediately following exposure to an allergen. A late stage response, happening when inflammatory cells have been brought in for backup, can occur several hours after exposure. Allergic reactions can trigger hives in the skin's surface.

Usually hives are seen on the arms, legs, and chest, but they might occur on different areas of the human body. A serious allergic response, like the one our kid experienced, may cause swelling inside the mouth and throat.

Identifying Hives

Normal hives seen on the top layer of the skin appear as red lumps (welts). Many times, they're accompanied with itching and general distress, such as burning or stinging. They vary in size anywhere between involving a portion of an inch to the size of a little dish.

Even though welts are a common occurrence, they're not necessarily an indication of an allergic response.

When someone does break out in hives, they generally appear on a single portion of their human body then it spreads quite quickly to other areas. It is not strange for the welts to develop bigger and unite with different hives (or welts). Sometimes these welts can enlarge over huge surfaces of skin. The spreading of these hives can lead to senses such as shivering, burning off and extreme itching. The welts could appear and vanish, then reappear within the course a couple of minutes or a couple of days. Hives are related to allergic reactions to a lot of types of allergens, such as those related to food allergies.

Common signs of food allergies

Hives are among those I have discovered through my research which specific foods can trigger an assortment of issues. As we've seen, there's a link between inflammation and many disorders, ailments and food allergies, and a lot are linked to gluten.

As we've only discovered, there are lots of substances that could prompt an allergic response.

What I found essential is to be aware that milk and gluten trigger a couple of the most typical food allergies that highlight the benefits of a gluten free, milk free, diet plan!

Let me elaborate. A food allergy is brought on by the immune-system's reaction to

certain proteins found in meals. A number of symptoms may result in a runny nose, coughing, nausea, stomach aches and anaphylaxis (a very serious illness that occurs immediately, sometimes leading to death).

And if that is not enough, this response could possibly occur at any moment.

Allergic reactions might have anywhere between a really slight to a significant reaction. Whenever the food has been absorbed, certain radicals might be triggered that may bind together with all the food particles and provoke an autoimmune-inflammatory response. As we've discovered, inflammation of any sort can hinder the body's capacity to heal and enhance food correctly. Furthermore, these foods allergens are ordinarily not properly digested and develop in the liver, gut therefore, and every one the organs which are connected with, detox in the entire body. After removing glutens in their daily diet, a lot of individuals no longer experience allergic reactions to foods. The typical symptoms include those we've identified.

The immune system, allergies and stress

The impact of pressure on our system may cause several negative reactions. Our strategies have the built-in capability to deal with stress. Anxiety triggers a sudden rise in vitality, which is caused by stimulation from the stress hormone cortisol. Within our exceptionally stressful universe, this reaction could be actuated at any moment, even while sitting in rush hour traffic. The sudden burst of electricity permits for 'flight or fight', yet all this time we do not have the chance to utilize this greater energy. Since we don't have any way to utilize the blood glucose, we're frequently left with continuously elevated levels of cortisol. This prolonged elevation may weaken the immune system, increase the odds of allergic reactions, nausea, and raise the danger of several stress related health issues.

The harm of persistent use of allergic medicine

Over utilization of any medicine to counteract inflammatory responses includes particular dangers. In the instance of both anti-inflammatories, the dangers include cardiovascular difficulties, erectile disorder, gastrointestinal issues, inflammatory bowel disease, renal troubles and problems during pregnancy.

Because of this increased usage of anti-inflammatories, the unwanted ramifications are now progressively worse. The key adverse reactions include esophageal and gastrointestinal impairment. The side-effects may include nausea, gastrointestinal distress, and the danger of departure. Note

CHAPTER FOUR

The Benefits of Anti-Inflammatory Foods

Lately, inflammation has turned into a blasting point at the front line of wellbeing and health. It is one of the main sources of maturing and malady, nonetheless, much of the time, it is preventable. Our cutting-edge ways of life where we progressively experience the ill effects of interminable pressure, rest less hours than our bodies need, and consume less calories which leads to poor health in anti-inflammation supplements, have prompted constant aggravation in the body.

On a positive note, so as to counteract ceaseless irritation in the body, we can pursue an anti-inflammatory diet that helps keep the resistant framework solid, balance weight and keep all the body's framework working.

What does the anti-inflammatory diet comprise of?

This eating regimen centers around wiping out the nourishments that cause fiery reactions in the body, similar to gluten, dairy, sugar and handled foods, and trading them for wholefoods, for example, vegetables, entire grains, fish and natural products.

The foods most extravagant in anti-inflammatory nutrients you ought to incorporate into your eating routine are:

• Green verdant greens, for example, spinach and kale

• Celery

• Coconut oil

• Turmeric

• Ginger

• Chia Seeds

• Beetroot

• Broccoli

• Blueberries

• Salmon

• Walnuts

As should be obvious, they are meals that are anything but difficult to consolidate into your eating regimen every day. They will counteract untimely maturing and ailments, improve subjective capacity, reinforce the resistant framework and lift vitality levels. Lift your wellbeing and essentialness with the calming diet!

In contrast to the ordinary eating routine, it doesn't have a snappy name nor does it guarantee you'll drop a size by Saturday. It's not even an extreme eating regimen, in essence, however really it's an eating plan that wil stay with you forever. It's the alleged calming diet, or rather, the anti-inflammatory slims down. About at least six eating routine books depend on the calming thought and various web destinations call it "mitigating" eating.

The anti-inflammatory diet is perfect for great wellbeing. Defenders of the eating routine state it can lessen coronary illness hazard, hold existing heart issues under tight restraints, diminish blood triglycerides and circulatory strain, and calm delicate and hardened ligament joints. In any case, specialists yield that enemy of aggravation eating is more compelling for some medical issues than others,and that the logical proof for the malady decrease advantages of these eating plans is as yet being assembled.

Anti-inflammatory Diets: What Do You Eat?

People differ from eating routines to slim down, yet when all is said and done, mitigating diets recommend:

• Eat a lot of foods grown from the ground

• Minimize immersed and trans fats

• Eat a decent, wellspring of omega-3, unsaturated fats such as fish, fish oil enhancements and pecans

• Watch your admission of refined starches like pasta and white rice

• Eat a lot of entire grains such as dark colored rice and bulgur wheat

• Eat lean protein sources likechicken; cut back on red meat and full-fat dairy meals

• Avoid refined nourishments and prepared foods

• Spice it up. Ginger, curry and different flavors can have a calming impact.

As one case of anti-inflammatory eating, a morning meal could consist of toasted steel-cut oats with berries, yogurt, or other fixing and espresso or green tea. Lunch could be fish serving of mixed greens on 7-grain bread and a smoothie with occasional natural products. For a tidbit, attempt an ounce of dull chocolate and around four pecans. Supper could be spaghetti with turkey meat sauce, spinach serving of mixed greens with oranges and pecans, and apple cranberry pie made without spread.

"The eating regimens don't guarantee weight reduction, yet weight decrease does frequently happen. What's more, that bodes well, given the cosmetics of the eating routine," says Greenfield.

"When you are looking at curtailing red meat, dairy, fats and trans fats, halfway hydrogenated oils, profoundly handled carbs–and eating more beneficial protein like fish, eating more products of the soil–chances are that individuals will lose in any event a smidgen of weight."

Nourishment high in omega-6: omega-3 proportion

With an end goal to decrease irritation, it is suggested that you stay away from nourishments that have a high proportion of Omega-6 to Omega-3. Coming up next is a rundown of some basic sustenance that will, in general, have a high proportion.

1. Grains - 20:1

2. Seed and seed oils - 70:1

3. Soybean oil - 7:1

4. Chicken - 15:1

5. Potato Chips - 60:1

Advantages of omega-3

The long-chain types of omega-3 greasy acids are DHA and EPA. DHA is the structure square of cerebrum tissue and EPA is its forerunner. Next is a rundown of the advantages and conditions that are improved with omega-3 acids in the eating routine.

1. Healthier, more grounded bones

2. Improved state of mind guideline

3. Reduced danger of Parkinson's

4. Reduced danger of death from ALL causes

5. Prevention of vascular difficulties from Type-II diabetes

6. Gallstones

7. Multiple Sclerosis

8. Brain and eye improvement in children

9. Peripheral corridor sickness

10. Preventing post birth anxiety

11. Combating malignant growth

Foods high in omega-3

1. Flax seed oil

2. Canola oil

3. Walnuts

4. Fish

5. Shellfish

6. Krill

7. Cod liver oil

8. Omega-3 enhanced eggs

9. Pasture-raised meats

10. Wild rice

11. Beans

Anti-inflammatory foods

Alongside concentrating on nourishments that will give the right proportion of omega-6 to omega-3 unsaturated fats, there are likewise sure sustenance that have mitigating properties:

1. Vegetables

2. Fruit

3. Sweet potatoes and different tubers

4. Dark chocolate

5. Red wine

6. Coffee and tea

7. Ginger, turmeric, garlic and different flavors

8. Olive oil, coconut oil and spread

A quality fish oil supplement should be in your eating regimen. It's imperative to search for fish oil that has been molecularly refined and contains in any event 500 mg of both DHA and EPA. There are a lot of fish oil supplements available that will promote 1000 mg of fish oil, yet not all contain the suggested measure of those two acids.

The anti-inflammatory diet isn't generally an eating regimen; it's a greater amount of an eating plan. Furthermore, and when you do inquire about it a little, you'll see that there's not only one calming diet; there are a few, each with an alternate turn. For our motivations here, I've attempted to show what a 'nonexclusive' adaptation is. This form shares with the others the idea that proceeded and wild irritation prompts ailment, and that following an eating plan that abstains from aggravating the body advances wellbeing and can help forestall ailment.

As a rule a mitigating diet incorporates:

• Plenty of foods grown from the ground

• Plenty of entire grains (e.g., darker rice, bulgur wheat)

• Lean protein (e.g., chicken, fish)

• Anti-fiery flavors (e.g., curry, ginger)

• Omega-3 unsaturated fats, (for example, those found in fish, fish oil enhancements, and pecans)

• A decrease in:

- Refined starches (e.g., pasta, white rice)

- Red meat and full-fat dairy nourishments

- Saturated and trans fats

• No refined or handled foods

A few words of alert in regards to this arrangement: the impacts you experience (i.e., an improvement in your indications) won't be as quick as they would be in the event that you treated yourself with prescriptions. You most likely need to give the calming diet, in any event, two weeks versus the hour or two a prescription may take. On the opposite side, this eating routine may have a reward impact not generally found in prescriptions: weight reduction!

The easiest changes to boost health–Anti-inflammatory diet

There are a million and one stylish eating regimens out there offering to change what you look like and feel within a few days. The purchaser is overflowed with items that will cause their skin 'to show up' more advantageous and milder to contact. In a world with an excess of spotlight on looking great and 'showing up' more advantageous, there is one eating routine that will make you more beneficial and possibly carry on with a more drawn out life in your enemy of matured body.

The anti-inflammatory diet has such a large number of employments today it is astounding all of the wellbeing, wellness and magnificence masters have not hopped on the most straightforward of eating routine changes and promoted them as the following huge pattern in weight reduction, excellence and hostility matures. The truth of the matter is the calming diet can do everything other eating regimens guarantee they can do and build life expectancy all the while.

The benefits of natural anti-inflammatory these days

Regular enemy of inflammatory are prudent, and individuals are currently much better instructed in what is great and terrible for them. Clearly setting off to the burger bar every day, or eating gigantic amounts of nourishment is awful for you, and ought to be kept away from. Probably the most straightforward approaches to ease torment brought about by irritation is to pursue an eating routine dependent on characteristic enemy of inflammatory. This implies eating more products of the soil, fish and chicken, while eliminating bread, intemperate sugar, starches and prepared or bundled nourishment.

Omega-3 unsaturated fats repress the action of the catalysts that crush the ligament tissues in the joints. They normally decrease aggravation and lessen torment. Fish is one of the better wellsprings of omega-3, and ought to be eaten consistently. A standard measurement of omega-3 as unadulterated fish oil enhancements is fantastic for excited joints.

What we should take a look at are regular cures given by such things as turmeric, ginger, rosemary and green tea. These are, for the most part, characteristic enemy of inflammatory items that decreases swelling in joints. Dull verdant greens, avocados and pecans can be eaten consistently, and healthful oils such as evening primrose, can be accepted day by day as enhancement.

Just as what we ought to eat, there is an entire host of nourishments we ought to stay away from. We should constrain our admission of red meat, dairy items and immersed fats. We should cook nourishments with olive oil rather than vegetable oil and cut down on creature proteins. Eating bunches of fiber that are found in leafy foods is additionally prescribed, as is drinking tea as opposed to espresso. It is additionally prudent to drink up to eight glasses of water every day.

Adjacent to that, an eating routine dependent on the common enemy of inflammatory is generally utilized and accepted to have the option to help keep your wellbeing to stay ideal and furthermore influence the recuperating procedure of individuals who have endless inflammation issues.

Common anti-inflammatory foods for better health and less pain

Inflammation is due to distress, swelling, warmth and redness around the affected kingdom. There is an assortment of options to take care of inflammation. One can be prescriptions, which thus far has not been greatest because it does not generally repair the matter. Another alternative is the standard manner, from wherever our entire body starts out of; our own body been created ordinarily and has its routine items from character.

This means choosing the nutrition your body requires, because deficiencies of particular fixings no doubt resulted in the illness whatever the instance. It's understood our body is able to react to nourishments, because particular sustenance being used vary to other men and women. What that suggests, as in annoyance, is a couple of sustenance may really have a positive or negative effect. Listed below is a section of the normal calming nourishments; if selected effectively, they'll have that impact in recovering.

Normal anti-inflammatory foods

Vegetables and organic goods: blossoms, goods of green and fabulous shading assist the process of fiery ailments. Vegetables and organic goods are full of mobile reinforcements, by way of instance, nutrients, fiber and minerals that the body requires daily to stay sound. These have cancer prevention representatives, phytochemicals and anti-inflammatory possessions present.

Significant fats

Likewise, rich in anti-inflammatory nourishments are olive oil, coconut oil, lettuce and avocados. Each of these include omega-3, polyunsaturated fats that are essential for joint and swelling health. The corrosive in omega-3 is a provocative operator which transforms into prostaglandins that's a hormone-like material. Omega-3 is not beneficial for joint distress and aggravation. We simply acquire omega out of our eating regime, thus it's critical to incorporate some of the strong oils such as olive, macadamia and krill, that can be much more pliable than fish oil. There are many options of sustenance available which comprise a range of omega.

Oils you should think about

Jojoba oil has significantly more medical benefits that many folks don't figure out. Create a point to use it on your eating regime. Olive oil is full of cancer prevention representatives and comprises of a chemical known as oleuropein. Medicinal science has verified that additional virgin olive oil is perhaps the most advantageous sustenance we can add to our eating routine.

This oil is most useful and viable for joint inflammation sufferers since it can cool inflammation and simplify joint torment. Be that as it may, for cooking, searing, heating and so on, utilize just coconut or macadamia nut oil. Different oils when warmed become lethal, and more often than not, transform into trans fats which can trigger irritation and joint torment, as well as other medical problems. Keep a strategic space for these types of oils: citrus oils, including soy bean and canola. These would be the typical ones that the huge majority consider in light of these titles. Really, they have a strong sounding title, nevertheless they aren't beneficial.

Flavors

Turmeric will be within the rundown in reducing inflammation and joint distress. Additionally, garlic includes a chemical curcumin that's famous for several medical benefits and has the capability to mend joint distress. It's best used in its own feature. Adding it to your own eating routine when possible, the longer the better. Other vital flavors used for decreasing inflammation include cinnamon, garlic, rosemary, peppermint and ginger. All these are packed with antioxidants and bioflavonoids that help to reduce irritation and ward off free radicals. Cayenne pepper is also famous for its mitigating home and its own capsicum material that's added to specific creams for assistance with distress.

Grains

Whole grains that contain starches can similarly help in preventing spikes from the glucose level of their blood, because it recognizes that inflammation. Whatever the scenario, use just non-refined whole grains, even when planning has happened and all of the integrity is missing, for instance, nutrients, fiber and minerals. One of the top grains comprise oats: complete wheat, whole wheat, quinoa, couscous and bulgar. To choose a multi nutritional supplement for beneficial purposes, it may fill the place of specific food you normally may not gain from the eating regimen as required daily. Whatever the case, your initial need should always function as eating regime, only when choosing an improvement, you'll get the greatest esteem.

Eating anti-inflammatory herbs and diets

I've carried out much research on irritation, how it influences our ways of life and the nature of living. Eating anti-inflammatory diet and herbs is by all accounts a larger method for expanding the nature of an individual's life over a significant amount of time. In the present day and age, individuals are living longer than at any other time, yet is the nature of that life improving as well?

One needs to ask themselves the inquiry, is it extremely beneficial to live till I'm 90 if the most recent 15 years of my life are loaded up with things as alzheimer chemotherapy and joint pain? It appears that despite the fact that individuals are living longer and more, the measure of sicknesses and afflictions present in the cutting-edge world appear to be on the ascent too.

A major reason for this is the eating regimens of what we eat. Anybody would contend that the standard diet is loaded up with sustenance and that much of it isn't generally solid. The sheer volume of additives, fake hues and sugars, pesticides, prepared nourishments and different things in the diet is really amazing. A great part of the diet appears to realize a general condition of irritation happens inside the body. Irritation as an idea is an fantastic thing, shielding areas of our bodies from unsafe and perilous things. Inflammation happens when an individual gets bit by a noxious bug, or when an abrupt effect causes a gruff power injury to a specific locale of the body. By swelling and separating the district, the body can best shield itself from further mischief and find a way to fix the harm.

An issue happens when the body empowers toward an expert provocative state through the utilization of specific sustenance. Diets by and large are said to either be inflammatory or star provocative. As you can envision, sustenance that are master incendiary will expand the measure of inflammation an individual encounters in different pieces of their body. Torment will for the most part increment, and the danger of numerous endless illnesses appears to rise. Sustenance like low quality nourishments, quick nourishments, sugar, handled sustenance and high fat meats are at the highest priority on the rundown of anti-inflammatory nourishments. As an individual's body goes into a raised condition of inflammation, comparing diseases like joint inflammation, appear to develop extraordinary and are increasingly agonizing too.

Expending nourishments advancing a calming state appears to positively affect an individual's wellbeing and health as time goes on. There is a great deal of writing that has just been expounded on anti-inflammatory diets and anybody inspired by the theme should keep doing research regarding the matter. I first began inquiring about the theme when I was made mindful of the joint pain that keeps running in my family. I needed to check whether there was anything I could do that would help stop the joint pain before it began. That carried me to inquiring about anti-inflammatory nourishments and herbs. I found that all in all, to keep an attitude of staying away from nourishments that caused inflammation in the body, would prompt a general condition of health and would enable the body to battle interminable ailments like joint pain. So as it were, having a legacy of joint inflammation in my family was a gift since it drove me to look into approaches about how to improve my general wellbeing. Anti-inflammatory herbs and diets are certainly something that merits thought.

How Inflammation Triggers Diabetes—And Anti-Inflammatory Tips to Live By

Inflammation is rising as a key factor hidden in the advancement of type 2 diabetes, and it's one that numerous individuals have not known about. A typical and totally common body reaction, inflammation is a procedure by which your white platelets and body synthetic substances shield you from microorganisms, infections and disease.

You can identify intense inflammation in your body by redness, warmth, swelling and torment at the site of damage. These are signs that your body is effectively battling a contamination.

In any case, under numerous conditions–regularly because of the way of life factors or an over-responsive resistant framework–inflammation can be endless, prompting a poor-quality condition of decay in your body. For this situation, inflammation causes no apparently indications despite the fact that it might harm your framework, which is the reason it's otherwise called 'quiet' inflammation.

Constant 'quiet' inflammation isn't just embroiled in ceaseless infections like coronary illness, malignancy, Alzheimer's malady and rheumatoid joint inflammation, yet additionally in type 2 diabetes.

Your Diet and Your Lifestyle Habits Can Increase Inflammation Too

Numerous variables can invigorate incessant inflammation in your body, including:

1. Overweight and corpulence

2. Unhealthy eating routine

3. Poorly controlled diabetes

4. Lack of activity

5. Gum sickness

6. Smoking

7. Stress

8. Long-term contaminations

You will see that numerous things on this rundown–unhealthy eating regimen, absence of activity, gum ailment–will place increments into your type 2 diabetes hazard, so when you need to stay away from diabetes, it's critical to find a way to decrease the inflammation in your body.

This incorporates:

• Avoid expert inflammatory foods. The following nourishments may add to foundational inflammation: trans fats (found in mostly hydrogenated vegetable oil), singed sustenance, sugar, bread and other refined carbs, soft drink, liquor and polyunsaturated vegetable oils.

• Eating a lot of calming foods. Foods that help diminish inflammation incorporate crisp products of the soil and wild-got fish (for the omega-3 fats).

• Exercising

• Quitting smoking

• Reducing worry in your life

• Considering certain calming herbs and flavors, for example, turmeric, ginger and boswellia.

It's critical to downplay constant irritation in your body to decrease your danger of type 2 diabetes as well as various other endless sicknesses.

How would you know whether you have chronic inflammation?

The C-Reactive Protein (CRP) test is the most widely recognized test used to distinguish inflammation; it gauges a protein in your body that increments during fundamental inflammation. In one investigation, ladies with raised CRP levels were observed to be almost multiple times bound to create diabetes than those with lower levels, and even in the wake of modifying for other hazard factors, the hazard was still more than multiple times as high.

Nonetheless, regardless of whether you realize you have raised CRP levels or not, it's a smart thought to make the strides above to decrease inflammation in your body. We are all affected by inflammation to a certain degree, and the best alternative to keep the perpetual, diabetes-connected sort away is to lead a sound way of life as depicted previously.

You may likewise consider fish oil supplements which can be extremely high in omega-3 unsaturated fats, which have appeared in research concentrates to go about as an anti-inflammation, and accordingly diminishes your danger of cardiovascular illness and different ailments. Omega-3 fish oil unsaturated fats, especially EPA, have a constructive outcome on your provocative reaction. By helping the body produce anti-inflammatory eicosanoids, omega-3 unsaturated fats help your body control it's inflammation cycle, which avoids and alleviates difficult conditions and ailment. For grown-ups, fish oil supplements with omega-3 improve memory, review, thinking just as center and fixation.

Magnesium is a Powerful Natural Anti-Inflammatory Mineral

While magnesium has consistently been known to be an extremely incredible mineral, another investigation, including 3,713 postmenopausal ladies, has completely demonstrated its anti-inflammatory impacts. With 100 mg of magnesium for every day, anti-inflammatory properties were experienced. Magnesium could be of extraordinary guide to the individuals who wish to stay away from the awful reactions of anti-inflammatory pharmaceuticals.

As per the investigation, inflammatory markers, for example, CRP (C-responsive protein), TNFa (tumor rot factor alpha), and IL6 (interleukin 6), were altogether diminished when magnesium admission was expanded. This implies magnesium assumes an immediate job in bringing down basic provocative markers, which further demonstrates its helpful properties.

Inflammation has been attached to endless ailments and makes millions of people to endure it every day. Utilizing magnesium to help in the battle against inflammation is a savvy choice, and one that requires no pharmaceuticals.

Do you know about the Fish Oil Anti-Inflammation Diet?

Have you at any point pondered, for what reason why, media humming has such a great amount of hostility toward the inflammation diet? This is a direct result of the stunning finishes of numerous examinations on hindering inflammation in the body. Hyper-inflammation can be the main driver of numerous wellbeing concerns, running from minor ones like wrinkles, male pattern baldness and sensitivities to significant ones like heart assaults, disease, joint pain, and psoriasis etc.

An enemy of inflammation diet will bode well in the event that we comprehend, but what sustenance sources have inflammation impact and what does not have? At that point it will be simple for us to choose the inflammation free diet that we, as a whole, have been longing for.

Nuts, tofu, flaxseeds, ocean bottom creatures like fish, shrimps and clams are rich wellsprings of omega-3 unsaturated fats, while chicken, hamburger, pork and different oils like sunflower oil, hemp oil, pumpkin oil etc, are wealthy in omega-6 unsaturated fats.

As a result of our dietary patterns (we eat a great deal of slick, seared and lousy nourishment), a large portion of us have elevated amounts of omega-6 fats (they have irritation property) and are insufficient in omega-3 fats. The perfect proportion of omega-6 to omega-3 for a sound body is 4:1, however much of the time, it is as high as 50:1. Along these lines, we need an enemy of inflammation diet (omega-3 fats) to counteract the inflammation in the body.

Studies have demonstrated that DHA omega-3 fat can be changed over to a compound substance called resolvin D2. D2 is an awesome inflammation specialist. In this way sustenance sources that are rich in DHA ought to be incorporated into our every day diet routine to control the body's inflammation cycle.

Slick and cold-water fish, similar to wild salmon, hoki, halibut, mackerel, herring and sardines, are rich in DHA. In any case, due to the expanding contamination in the sea waters, fish will general gather poisons as well. Consequently, eating them routinely isn't suggested.

A simple choice is to take fish oil supplements. These enhancements experience the different refining procedures to sift through all the destructive poisons and synthetic concoctions like mercury, lead, arsenic, PCBs and so on. Accordingly, with their utilization, you can achieve wanted degrees of DHA and EPA with no stresses of polluting influences.

In one of the clinical preliminaries, it was seen that enhancements produced using the blend of hoki oil and fish oil have more than double the calming impact as in contrast with different enhancements. Unadulterated and high DHA fish oil supplement can go about as a powerful enemy of irritation diet. It, other than decreasing the soreness in your body, will likewise expand your future.

CHAPTER FIVE

What Can I Do To Reduce Inflammation In My Body?

What causes Inflammation in the body and how do I control it?

Inflammation in the body is really useful and is treated as a major aspect of the body's framework. It goes about as a layer between the external condition and the influenced territory; it also represses the disease to spread to other body parts. In the event that there is an occurrence of any damage or disease, we see redness and soreness around the influenced territory. This is on the grounds that; the WBCs (white platelets) are joined to the inward linings of veins around the influenced territory.

Then again, if due to any reason, if WBCs begin regarding solid cells as remote material, increasingly more of WBCs begin gathering at the internal linings, bringing about agony and overabundance of soreness. This outcomes in endless inflammation, which if not controlled at before, stages can prompt difficult conditions like arthritis, psoriasis etc.

In the wake of understanding what causes irritation, let us currently discover a successful method for controlling it.

The best and regular approach to have a tab on the body's irritation cycle is to accomplish elevated amounts of DHA omega-3 unsaturated fats. These are long chain polyunsaturated fats, which are required by the body for its legitimate development and improvement. Studies have demonstrated that the body can change over DHA to a synthetic called resolvin D2 that has a property to respond with internal linings of veins to shape nitric oxide. This layer of nitric oxide hinders abundance of WBCs to join the internal linings of veins, and thus helps in diminishing inflammation.

In this manner, it is our enthusiasm to have high DHA levels. Be that as it may, since the body can't deliver DHA alone, we need to take express activities to incorporate high DHA sustenance sources in our every day diet.

Cold-water fish like hoki, tuna, salmon, etc, are the rich wellspring of DHA fats. In any case, in view of expanding water contamination, fish are additionally loaded with pollutions like mercury, lead and arsenic. Clearly, it's anything but a decent arrangement to lessen inflammation in the body at the expense of eating poisons.

This is the place fish oil enhancements come to help. They experience refining procedures to expel all the undesirable and destructive synthetic compounds from the oil and are consequently, useful for human utilization.

Since you realize what causes inflammation in the body and how you can control the equivalent, your subsequent stage ought to be investing some more energy in the web to discover a viable enhancement and begin taking it right away.

Perpetual Inflammation in the body is dangerous

You know when you have a sore throat and your lymph hubs are swollen? Your body has sent in the military of white platelets to wreck the encompassing tissue and improve. The issue comes when it doesn't quit obliterating the sound tissue and continues onward.

Specialists have connected inflammation in your body with illnesses of different types such as asthma, rheumatoid joint pain, coronary illness, considerably malignant growth and memory misfortune.

Studies demonstrate it is basic to your wellbeing and prosperity to control inflammation in the body.

You may consider inflammation in swollen joints from joint pain agony or the swelling encompassing a paper cut, however, inflammation can be inside where its not obvious.

Excited corridors cause plaque development and block up the entry, which adds to a heart assault. Moreover, inflammation in your cerebrum blocks up the neuron pathways so the messages aren't clear or don't get sent–this can prompt Alzheimer's.

Inflammation begins as your body's barrier against damage or sickness. It's your body's method for mending you. However, when its work is done, the inflammation should stop. Chronic inflammation can cause long haul harm.

The guide to getting rid of Inflammation in your body

Many of us experience the ill effects of inflammation in our bodies and we should comprehend what inflammation truly is.

Inflammation is a procedure brought about by our bodies to shield us from unsafe diseases or infection. If you experience the ill effects of inflammation in your body, you will have encountered redness or torment. There are numerous reasons for inflammation. It can be intense or incessant, but whichever way, there are a few things that you can do to dispose of it. Along these lines, how about we begin examining how to lessen inflammation in the body.

Decreasing this issue in your body is certifiably not a troublesome assignment. So as to do this, you should watch what you eat and practice normally. How about we talk about each in detail.

When attempting to stay away from inflammation in your body; you should diminish your admission of handled nourishment. All and any sort of handled nourishment will contain sustenance that builds the irritation level in your body. Additionally, attempting to maintain a strategic distance from sustenance that contains high measures of sugar can consequentlyanticipate the issue that you should eat vegetables and organic products.

Vegetables and natural products contain mitigating properties. These nourishments have demonstrated to diminish irritation in the whole body. It is proposed to expend the vegetables and natural products that are brilliant in shading.

Additionally, in your customary eating diet increment, the admission of omega-3 unsaturated fat. Omega-3 is generally found in various kinds of nuts and seeds. Accordingly, make sure to eat pecans or sesame seeds all the time. Research demonstrates that green tea and straightforward water can help keep this issue from happening. Green tea and water are referred to go about as cell reinforcements, and with normal use, they will limit the issue. Aside from watching what you eat, practicing has demonstrated to help in keeping this from occurring. With exercise you will shed pounds, when you get in shape the measure of weight on your joints will be less. The less weight on your joints will help forestall an inflammation issue. Nonetheless, you should guarantee that you normally practice for in any event for 40 minutes.

The previously mentioned systems are best in assisting with inflammation in the body. In any case, you can take supplements which are wealthy in fish oil or nutrients. Alongside these enhancements, ordinary body back rubs have demonstrated to help in preventing this from occurring. These back rubs should be possible with oil or basic creams. You can keep warmed cushions on your body, which will absolutely help. Despite the fact that these methods work, they are not as compelling as the adjusting of the eating regimen and working out. In this way, when attempting to ensure the body, you ought to consistently select to control what you eat and practice normally. Keep in mind, that regardless of what procedure you pick, you have to guarantee that you are steady with it. Inflammation is treatable just in the event that you are given.

Step by step instructions to reduce Chronic Inflammation in your body

Joint inflammation, bursitis, tendonitis, plantar fasciitis, colitis, dermatitis, pancreatitis, appendicitis and sinusitis; what do these conditions share? They end with the inflammation in your framework. Once in a while inflammation is only a sign of abuse or mileage, yet in some cases, something in the resistant framework has gone astray, especially in regards to crippling incendiary issues. So how about we investigate the components that impact inflammation and either lose or keep the resistant framework on track.

1. **Food sensitivities** –In the rundown event that somebody is giving indications of an incendiary condition, they need to survey and expel nourishment hypersensitivities from their eating

regimen. Nearly everybody has sustenance sensitivities. In testing more than 500 patients, everyone except for three patients had nourishment hypersensitivities. The vast majority had no clue they did on the grounds that the indications of some sustenance sensitivities can be postponed and inconspicuous, a few out of every odd nourishment hypersensitivity, is as emotional or dangerous as a nut sensitivity. Sensitivities that are interceded by antibodies can cause such wide and changed manifestations as clogging, loose bowels, swelling, gas, sinus blockage, joint torment, cerebral pains, exhaustion, skin rashes, dermatitis, psoriasis, skin inflammation, sniffling, runny nose, watery eyes and irritated mouth/nose/ears. Eating something you are adversely affected by strains your invulnerable framework and incites inordinate irritation.

2. **The stomach related tract** –The abundance of unfortunate microscopic organisms, or yeast in the stomach related tract, can make a harmed/aroused stomach related tract. This implies that the invulnerable framework isn't working appropriately since 70-80% of your insusceptible framework is situated around your stomach related

tract. This unfortunate condition and conceivable absence of good microorganisms alludes to as a probiotic microscopic organism, and can create awkwardness in the resistant framework, which incites more inflammation. It makes the gut be progressively flawed, permitting inadequate stomach related nourishment section into the body where the insusceptible framework can experience it, creating more sustenance hypersensitivities and inflammation.

3. **Adrenal weariness or adrenal weakness –** Adrenals are your pressure organs. They help your body manage worry alongside numerous different capacities including: control circulatory strain, direct glucose, help with hormone balance that give you vitality, drive and inspiration.Corticosteroids are an amazing enemy of inflammatory pain. They are here and there, given as a medication to address incendiary conditions as prednisone or corticosteroid puffers or nasal splashes. Supporting your adrenal organs can fix the body's capacity to make it's own corticosteroids, diminishing the requirement for outside admission.

4. **Lack of Nutrient C and Nutrient B6** –Both are normal enemies of histamines. And when they get exhausted you will be increasingly inclined to hypersensitivities and the inflammation related with it.

5. **Lack of Omega-3 unsaturated fats** –Our eating regimens will in general be overwhelming in omega-6 unsaturated fats and proportionately light in omega3's. The most productive approach to get omega-3's is from fish oil, either through expending fish two to three times each week or by enhancing the body with fish oil.

6. **Obesity** –Aside from the way that being overweight puts an additional strain on the joints, ligaments and tendons, which can incite irritation of the joints, ligaments or tendons, heftiness itself causes a constant inflammation. This inflammation has been connected to the improvement of insulin obstruction and type 2 diabetes.

Presently, you can smother inflammation utilizing calming prescriptions such as NSAIDs or prednisone, yet these are regularly joined by huge dangers and reactions like draining stomach ulcers, expanded danger of heart assault, or stroke and osteoporosis. They don't address the basic reason for the inflammation. Fixing the basic reason assuages side effects on a progressively lasting premise, without the symptoms and enables your body to recuperate.

How to reduce Inflammation in the body that requires your attention

You're savvy to think about how to decrease inflammation in the body. What's more, you're significantly more astute to proceed to do it. All things considered; inflammation is the number reason for death. Time magazine called it "the Silent Killer" and specialists concur. Constant inflammation is the hidden explanation behind all intents and purposes for each savage malady you can consider.

Alright, so you realize you have to do it. How?

The means are basic, however difficult. It will require some move in your reasoning. Some way of life changes. In any case, is it certifiably not a more drawn out, more beneficial life justified, despite all the trouble?

Basic to decreasing your inflammation is your eating routine and exercise. In case you're eating a lousy nourishment, diet loaded up with refined flours and sugars, you're making inflammation in your body. At any rate restorative research demonstrates that is what's valid for the vast majority.

The manifestations of inflammation, swelling, redness and throbbing can be occurring inside your body without you knowing it. They're a sign your invulnerable framework is lopsided.

Supplanting undesirable nourishments with a lot of foods grown from the ground and getting ordinary exercise will help diminish inflammation for some individuals.

And when you presume a nourishment hypersensitivity/affectability, you can remove the potential sustenance for three times a month and check whether that makes a difference. A few specialists prescribe the 'Base Diet' where you only eat fish, meat, vegetables and organic products for a month. The thought is you're not eating any cutting edge handled sustenance including grains. For some, this might be your answer.

It is proper to say that you are interested in reducing Inflammation?

Decreasing inflammation is presumably the most significant dietary advance anybody can take. It is a two-stage process that isn't troublesome. Be that as it may, the arrangement must be reliable when you need your wellbeing to be steady.

Inflammation is the thing that happens when your insusceptible framework escapes balance. A significant number of the present greatest wellbeing concerns are connected to inflammation of the body–malignant growth, coronary illness, stomach related framework issues and cerebrum related issues.

On one hand, this lopsidedness is brought about by an excess of white breads, vegetable oils, dairy items and handled nourishments. Then again, the normal Westerner is just not getting enough of the omega-3 basic unsaturated fats found in fish oil.

Omega-3s are a characteristic calming that help a solid body do what can do. That is battling sickness or outside contaminants without over responding.

For example, specific sorts of joint pain are just inflammatory joints. The body has sent too many white platelets and synthetic substances to the joint zone. The swelling causes torment and firmness. Lessening irritation with omega-3s likewise diminishes the weight and can reestablish versatility.

Here is the issue. Over 90% of us don't get enough omega-3s. Indeed, we are off by a long shot. The FDA and others accept that 2-3g's of fish oil omega-3s every day are helpful for keeping up a sound grown up safe framework. The FDA additionally suggests a limit of two servings of fish for each week. Different specialists think even that is excessive.

This is the reason the fish oil supplement market is developing so quickly. It is incredibly hard to get a base dose through our weight control plans.

An ongoing report from Finland pursued 21,000 individuals for around 11 years. Individuals who reliably took about 250mg of omega-3 fish oil enhancements had a half decrease in cardiovascular infection over the individuals who did not. Notice that reliably taking even little dosages was fruitful in diminishing inflammation.

And when you are not kidding about lessening inflammation, your following stage is to examine the enhancement showcase. In nature, balance is everything. Begin the arrangement. You may get yourself more beneficial, less tranquilize subordinate and rationally progressively engaged. This sort of way of life can be addictive (and in a decent way).

Treatment for Inflammation—Diet alone isn't enough to reduce Inflammation

In the event that you do any measure of finding out about medications for inflammation, you will discover heaps of exhortation on dietary changes as a treatment for irritation. This is for the most part a word of wisdom.

In any case, in the event that you need to diminish irritation, you should accomplish more than roll out a couple of improvements to your eating regimen. While the suggested dietary changes are great and for the most part substantial, there is one extra thing that you have to totally diminish inflammation.

Myth #1: Reducing awful fats is sufficient...

Don't misunderstand me–decreasing the awful fats in your eating regimen is extraordinary guidance. In any case, if exhortation that you read persuades this is everything necessary, you are being deluded. Possibly not deliberately, yet this isn't the long and short of it.

Myth #2: Exercise and weight reduction is the key...

Once more, these are generally excellent things. We all ought to get a lot of activity and monitor our weight. Yet, in the event that you are persuaded this is the main treatment for inflammation, there is one extra thing that you should comprehend to lessen inflammation.

There is something many refer to as 'Inflammation Syndrome' and it impacts your typical inflammation reaction. Aggravation Syndrome is a perpetual condition that changes your typical inflammation reaction to damage or injury. Incessant aggravation is a period bomb and incredibly risky to your long haul wellbeing.

Fundamental inflammation is a noteworthy inconspicuous issue in the vast larger part of the populace. It is additionally called 'quiet inflammation' since it is sub-intense. As it were, it's inconspicuous and flies under the radar. However, it is in charge of an enormous host of chronic conditions. Fortunately, there are some straightforward answers. You can discover long haul alleviation and decrease inflammation that will demolish your wellbeing. Also, it's anything but difficult to do!

The best diet to reduce Inflammation in the body

So, you're searching for an eating routine to lessen inflammation in the body, they do exist. Nonetheless, do you know what the best diet is?

Whatever the eating regimen, in the event that it has a high omega-3 unsaturated fat substance and a low measure of omega-6, it will undoubtedly be powerful. Omega-6 give our body inflammation while omega-3 contains calming properties.

It is significant that we do get four-fold the amount of omega-6 than omega-3 in our eating routine to be solid. Be that as it may, as of late this proportion has developed to be lopsided.

Rather than being 4:1, we end up with a proportion of 20:1 or 40:1 between omega-6 and omega-3. This is the reason our eating regimens need little omega-6 and more omega-3 - to adjust this proportion.

This do as well, we have to locate the best wellspring of omega-3, as this will result in...

The best diet to reduce Inflammation in the body

The most normally rich source in omega-3 is fish. Greasy fish like fish, hoki, sardines, mackerel, salmon and trout contain large amounts of DHA and EPA, the two basic unsaturated fats.

Be that as it may, our waters are dirtied. This implies the fish we eat for the most part contains unsafe poisons like mercury, lead, arsenic, dioxins and PCBs.

These are harming to our wellbeing and subsequently ought to be evaded. Be that as it may, how would we get the decency of fish in a sheltered manner?

A fish supplement is the most ideal approach to diminish aggravation in the body. They can be decontaminated to be powerful and safe.

The best cleansing procedure is called atomic refining. Pay special mind to this term in the event that you start to explore for an amazing enhancement.

A diet to reduce Inflammation in the body–yes, you have control

With all the inflammation startles it's not a big surprise that many individuals are searching for an eating regimen to lessen irritation in the body. That is to say, specialists presently accept most, if not all, sickness starts with endless inflammation. What's more, you definitely know there's a rash of diseases, joint pain and auto invulnerable issue like lupus. Different investigations demonstrate that hidden in each of these is aggravation.

A study found a connection among aggravation and disease. What's more, others have found connects to diabetes, asthma, hypersensitivities and each other ailment you can name.

Luckily, you can take care of business. Exercise, rest and an inspirational disposition will all assistance and lessen irritation. Dietary changes will help with this as well.

Flavors and Herbs

Rosemary, turmeric and ginger all have calming properties. Actually, ginger has been perceived as a characteristic irritation reducer for 1000's of years. In this way, add more to your fish and chicken.

Fish

Talking about fish, it's perhaps the best sustenance to incorporate into your eating routine to decrease irritation. Fish are wealthy in omega-3 unsaturated fats, which are important for irritation decrease. That is the reason your PCP proposes you eat more fish or take fish oil supplements. Fish is rich in DHA and EPA which are building hinders for your mind so they ensure your memory. The EPA keeps your state of mind adjusted so you remain increasingly positive.

That is the reason fish oil enhancements are so well known. They're advantageous, economical and can be filtered. Eating fish alone will give you about 30% of the omega-3 unsaturated fats you need. A decent quality fish oil supplement can give you 60% or more.

And when you pick an enhancement, make sure you get one with abnormal amounts of DHA and EPA. You likewise need to ensure they're sanitized utilizing a sub-atomic refining process. No compelling reason to ingest mercury and different poisons with your enhancements!

Best Natural remedy for Inflammation–reduce Inflammation in your body with Omega-3 Fish Oil

Is it true that you are searching for a successful characteristic solution for irritation? Omega-3 is a fundamental supplement that our bodies need to work; tragically the human body does not contain what is expected to make it. Along these lines, we can get it from our nourishments and by supplementation.

Inflammation is a guarded system utilized by the human body to fend off illnesses; along these lines, it is a characteristic event. In any case, a lot of it in your body prompts genuine medical issues like coronary illness, eye issue, joint pain and malignant growth; truth be told, it demonstrates that dominant part of ailments that are brought about by incessant inflammation.

Utilizing a characteristic solution for inflammation, for example, omega-3 fish oil is superior to anything taking NSAIDs like aspirin; the greater part of the NSAIDs have negative symptoms since they contain synthetic compounds that are unsafe to your body. Omega-3 contains DHA unsaturated fat, which is transformed into an amazing anti-inflammation operator known as resolvin D2.

In this way, and when you truly need a viable characteristic solution for aggravation, you should search for a fish oil supplement that contains high measure of DHA; the suggested least amount is 250 mg of DHA in a 1000mg case.

DHA lifts cerebrum capacities, learning, focus and memory; henceforth, it forestalls dementia and improves the states of those with other mind related issues like discouragement, ADD and mental imbalance.

The greater part of the omega-3 fish oil supplements available contain poisons such as mercury and PCBs; in this way, guarantee you purchase a brand that is purged by atomic refining. That is the main way you can make sure that you are taking unadulterated and safe oil.

Lessen Inflammation in two steps

Irritation in our body can cause:

- Acne, eczema and rosacea

- Food hypersensitivities and prejudices

- Digestive issues: IBS, colitis, Crohn's infection and candida

- Chronic weariness, fibromyalgia and general absence of vitality

- Brain mist, lack of focus and depression

- Attention shortage issue, poor learning and osmosis

- Sinus issues, chest diseases and asthma

- Dental issues, gum ailment

- Joint torment, back torment, muscle throbs, lupus and arthritis

- Thyroid brokenness

- Insomnia

- Weight gain, obesity

• And substantially more...

Given the rundown above (which is in no way, shape or form is complete), it makes sense that by controlling the incendiary reaction in the body and diminishing inflammation, we can improve our body. Consider when your brain is clear, you have huge amounts of vitality, your stomach feels light, your skin is gleaming, you are expressive and certainly free of agony, and you have a feeling that you can overcome the world. That is not a perfect world. It could be your existence once you are equipped with comprehension and inspiration to accomplish a more joyful variant of yourself.

To control inflammation, we have to comprehend what's causing it. Though the components adding to aggravation appear to be intricate, the fundamental points are: stomach related wellbeing and emotional wellbeing.

Inflammation can be brought about by:

1. Poor absorption, digestion and end

2. Mental and enthusiastic pressure

The Cerebrum Gut Association

Critically, the primary driver of inflammation (stomach related and mental) are really related. Our cerebrum registers musings. Each time an idea is enlisted, the mind makes a substance (a neuro-peptide) that is discharged into the blood. The small digestive tract does the very same thing, it produces the equivalent neuro-peptides, with the exception of in amounts multiple times more noteworthy contrasted with the cerebrum.

The neuro-peptides, once in the blood, work as a medication. When we engage glad musings (of appreciation, love, connectedness), we discharge upbeat synthetic substances (endorphins) from the mind and from the gut. These cheerful synthetics make us feel glad and turn on the various solid qualities. Then again, when we have troubled considerations, the cerebrum and the gut make destructive synthetics can turn on malignant growth qualities and trigger irritation, in addition to other things.

How to decrease irritation?

Right off the bat, deal with your feelings of anxiety:

1. Use reflection and supplication. Remember to favor your sustenance and water

2. Laugh more, observe more comedies and don't pay attention to yourself or life as well

3. Don't immerse yourself with an excess of savagery and 'fate and despair' circled by the media

4. Live with trustworthiness (lying or not satisfying your guarantees is in reality distressing, regardless of whether you deliberately acknowledge it or not)

5. Write an appreciation list day by day

6. Exercise consistently

7. Volunteer your time, ability, money or some other asset you may have for the benefit of other people. Commitment is probably the most noteworthy type of satisfaction and puts the body and mind into a mending state

8. Consider BodyTalk or other type of treatment to help you in cutting the worry down

Furthermore, yet similarly significant, get it together and tidy up your gut.

You are what you think and what you eat. The physical and the psychological go together, so you should address both. Here are a few things to support the stomach related framework, and accordingly, turn off aggravation:

1. Stay hydrated (this additionally causes you to release stuck feelings). Drink a glass of water 30 min before a feast. This can enable the stomach to process your nourishment better (and you will be processing your contemplations better, since the stomach meridian houses the cognizant personality)

2. Use flavors to support assimilation and cut down inflammation levels: turmeric (my top pick!), dark pepper, long pepper, cumin, fennel, coriander, ocean salt, Himalayan salt, ginger, cinnamon and cardamom are for the most part extraordinary when utilized with some restraint

3. Think about including some Ayurvedic supplements: Trikatu (helps stomach assimilation); Neem (helps clean and reestablish the small

digestive system, sanitizes blood and clears skin break out); Triphala (helps disposal from the internal organ, incredible for the eyes also); Boswellia (mends the coating of the small digestive tract and is extraordinary for decreasing generally speaking aggravation)

4. Incorporate nourishments that help reestablish the stomach related capacities: Lemon, coconut oil, ghee, chia seeds, linseeds, green vegetables, spirulina, beetroot, kumara, probiotic (non-improved) yogurts and kefir, slick fish

5. Eat organic products independently from different nourishments. Organic products, when joined with other nourishment, mature rapidly in the stomach and lead to gas, swelling, acid reflux, candida and aggravation

6. Some nutrients and minerals are significant for stomach related just as for emotional wellness: vitamin D, nutrient C, nutrient B complex, zinc. A decent probiotic supplement alongside basic unsaturated fats can help as well

7. Avoid espresso, liquor, sugar, prepared sustenance, nourishment added substances, refined carbs, hazardous fats. These sustenances are genius incendiary

8. Consider acquiring a customized nourishing counsel from a certified professional

Four effective Anti-Inflammatory herbs to reduce Inflammation

A few medications, steroids or herbs are known to have calming properties. In any case, what does calming imply? Inflammation is an intricate response of the body to the hurtful stimulant as aggravations, harmed cells or pathogens. Creatures attempt to shield itself from the stimulant, expels it and after that, it begins the recuperating procedure. This procedure is significant in light of the fact that injuries start to mend by virtue of this provocative response. Thus, those substances, as referenced before, have unique properties which speed-up the recuperating procedure and hence, are known as anti-inflammation.

At the point when inflammation starts, white platelets become dynamic, as their fundamental capacity is to fix and shield your life form from remote bodies, infections, microbes and so forth. White platelets have exceptional synthetic substances, which go to the kindled piece of the body and start to swell. In the event that the inflammation happens very close to the skin, that region winds up red in shading, warm and throbs, and additionally, blood stream increments. Agony is the most widely recognized indication of inflammation. In some cases, inward organs may get influenced excessively because of inflammation.

Valuable herbs: usually medications are the most well-known forms for treating inflammation, yet herbs may help you in an increasingly common and safe way. They diminish indications and make you feel much improved and they have extra helpful properties. So we should view the valuable herbs with anti-inflammation properties.

1. Turmeric: This is probably the best herb which viably fixes irritation like joint pain, auto-safe issue and tendonitis. Be that as it may, it won't work in a compelling way in the event that you are utilizing drugs. The greater part of the home grown cures need time. Be cautious and don't utilize turmeric regularly as it might cause indigestion. Pregnant women initially ought to counsel the specialist in the event that they need to utilize this herb.

2. Boswellia: It is broadly utilized in Ayurvedic drugs. Boswellia soothes the undesirable manifestations of inflammation being wealthy in normal properties, which are like the mitigating drugs. Interestingly, this herb does not bother the stomach related tract, and you can utilize it securely.

3. Ginger: Using ginger to ease the inflammation side effects is extremely valuable. This root is known to have numerous important properties. Likewise with turmeric, you should sit tight for quite a while for observable impact, yet the utilization of ginger is extremely worth pausing.

4. Licorice: You may also have a go at utilizing this herb. It is exceptionally compelling. Simply have it at the top of the priority list, so that you don't utilize it for exceptionally long times as it might cause potassium misfortune and hypertension.

There are a lot of increasingly home-grown cures, which can assist you with reducing inflammation. Arnica, fallen angels hook, bromelain, white willow and papaya should help you a great deal as well, however utilize every one of these herbs shrewdly and make sure that you are not sensitive to them. When you are sick with some other sickness, you better check with your primary care physician.

Keep up a solid way of life and eat legitimate nourishments and when you would prefer not to get into this condition. Treat every one of the maladies cautiously in order to maintain a strategic distance from further complexities.

Lessening Inflammation–The less Inflammation you have is better for your health

Inflammation is a procedure inside our very own bodies which is used to shield us from malady and damage. Like every one of these things throughout everyday life, a great deal can be terrible for us all. Any nutritionist or wellbeing mentor will educate you that the regular American eating regimen is topped off with nourishments which increment inflammation inside our very own bodies. These incorporate sugars, prepared grains and awful fats which are largely so common in most lousy nourishments. The issues associated with such an eating regimen are muscle or joint agony, asthma or sensitivities, higher pulse and glucose issues. This kind of eating regimen saps our vitality that you have to endure day by day.

A Healthier Diet to Lower Inflammation

And when you've been eating an eating regimen high in sugars, at that point you will sense a ton of advantages from the appropriation of an eating routine comprised of nourishments that diminish inflammation. The accompanying sorts of sustenance will help you in such a manner:

- Fruits

- Nuts

- Leafy green vegetables

- Fatty fish

- Fresh herbs and flavors

You may accomplish huge calming circumstances from removing fricasseed nourishments, soft drinks, prepared sugars and handled meats from your day to day diet. By adding the sound sustenance into your diet, the fat in fish and nuts can help feed your brain. Foods grown from the ground highlight loads of fundamental minerals and nutrients that help keep you sound while battling aggravation. At the point when combined with taking flavors and herbs, which are brimming with cancer prevention agents, you give your body precisely what it requires to feel the alleviation from the hurts, throbs, absence of vitality and different markers of a horrible eating routine.

You'll Thank Yourself

Altering your eating regimen is among the most troublesome prospects for some individuals. The vast majority of us catch wind of making New Year's goals, which are left a long time after, and wellness focus enrollments for those attempting to improve their wellbeing through exercise. You need to do anything that is required to roll out this improvement.

Teach yourself about sustenance on the web and through productions and eBooks, and furthermore consolidate gatherings on wellbeing related destinations and projects to connect with similar people that will help you to continue on. Should you require an exercise center coach to keep you on course, it may be the shrewdest venture you ever make. The mitigating advantages of a nutritious eating routine will give you the vitality and wellbeing to deal with your day by day existence with a force which you probably won't be able to imagine right now. When you have this capacity to carry on with the existence you constantly need, you won't ever need to come back to the manner that was you.

CHAPTER SIX
Classic Signs Of Inflammation

Inflammation is the body's organic reaction of endeavoring to secure itself. It means to expel unsafe boosts such as pathogens, harmed cells and inflammation; this is the initial step of the mending procedure. Inflammation triggers a reaction from the invulnerable framework, at first aggravation is gainful for insurance, however most times inflammation can prompt further aggravation.

The five signs to pay special mind to irritation are torment, redness, warmth, swelling and harmed work!

Chronic Inflammation

Chronic irritation is the point at which the underlying inflammation does not leave. It is never again a mending reaction, however it's a marker that something isn't right. Probably the greatest reason for incessant sickness originates from the nearness of 'perpetual incendiary status'. Ceaseless inflammation is long haul and can keep going for a considerable length of time or even years!

It is imperative to do all that you can to anticipate irritation so you don't arrive at this stage.

The provocative procedure is in charge of the indications and long haul harm connected with oxidative pressure.

Oxidative pressure happens when there is an excessive number of poisons for the body to manage. The body creates free radicals, and these harm the films of the cells, crushing significant proteins, fats and DNA.

Goals of an unending fiery condition lies at the core of all endeavors to treat and anticipate these horrible sicknesses.

There are a significant number of maladies and diseases which are brought about by interminable provocative conditions such as:

- Cardiovascular disease

- Diabetes type2

- Metabolic disorder

- Fibromyalgia

- Chronic exhaustion

- Depression

- Alzheimer's malady

- Cancer

- Osteoarthritis

- Ibs

- obesity

- atherosclerosis

Inflammatory conditions are regularly multifaceted

Cortisol–(testosterone is an enemy of inflammatory) is the most dominant enemy of inflammatory and is discharged in light of pressure (dhea is additionally an endogenous anti-inflammatory).

What causes the aggravation in any case?

- Chronic contaminations

- Obesity

- Environmental poisons (nourishment, water and air)

- Physiological pressure

- Intensive/aerobic exercise

- Physical injury

- Age

- Autoimmune sickness

Long haul pressure exacerbates any fiery condition.

What are the solutions?

If you are encountering the ill effects of interminable irritation, then it is imperative to diminish feelings of anxiety. Interminable inflammation is increasingly regular in overweight people, so one method for diminishing the odds of incessant inflammation is to pursue the standard methodology to losing muscle to fat ratio (good dieting and exercise).

Individuals' eating regimen should be improved to guarantee they are eating the majority of the essential nutrients and supplements while evading trans-fats and soaked fats. Eating herbs and flavors like turmeric, garlic, onions and a lot more are connected with lessening levels of irritation. The anti-inflammatory mixes found in these herbs and flavors give good wellbeing from numerous points of view.

Guarantee to get lots of rest and take enemies of oxidants. Those who are encountering the ill effects of endless inflammation do because of their way of life, so as to decrease their manifestations, then the way of life should be changed. Weight is a poor quality condition of incessant inflammation, so battling the fat will battle inflammation simultaneously!

As per the most recent restorative hypothesis, ceaseless irritation is the main driver of pretty much every infection endured by people. It's hard to believe, but it's true. Numerous specialists accept diligent, low-level inflammation prepares for unending illness, including those we normally experience late throughout everyday life like joint pain, heart and kidney illness, and disease.

As a piece of our safe reaction system, inflammation happens when the body is battling germs that enter the body through an assortment of ways, for example, damage or inward breath. When you experience redness, swelling, warmth, disease and agony from an assortment of infirmities, it's an indication of inflammation. Regularly, the inflammation leaves when the body has vanquished the disease or damage, however, when the body neglects to close off the inflammation procedure, an increasingly genuine condition can happen.

It is commonly perceived that heart assaults happen when the veins become stopped up with 'plaque' (what we more often than not alluded to as the awful LDL cholesterol) that is kept on the vessel dividers. This awful cholesterol gets inserted inside supply routes and our invulnerable framework 'assaults' it. Persevering irritation in the veins can in the end cause plaque to blast. Presently numerous specialists utilize a basic blood test for aggravation called CRP (short for C-Receptive Protein) to help survey an individual's cardiovascular hazard. CRP is a list of irritation in the supply routes and the CRP increments as aggravation increments. For instance, test have demonstrated that moderately aged men with high CRP levels in their blood were multiple times bound to endure a heart assault in the following six years than men with typical levels. Therapeutic specialists state that a CRP of 3.0 mg/L or higher triples your heart assault hazard. Individuals with CRP under 0.5 mg/L once in a while have heart assaults.

Fortunately we can plan something to decrease the dangers of constant inflammation, including getting in shape, practicing routinely and eating the correct diet. As indicated by the Center for Human Nutrition at Johns Hopkins School of Public Health, a few diets can cause aggravation while others can diminish it. Diets that are wealthy in leafy foods, and diets that offer heaps of omega-3 unsaturated fats, (such as salmon, fish, mackerel and pecans) are ideal. Further, an eating regimen of such nourishments has been demonstrated to be instrumental in weight decrease, and bringing down CRP and insulin opposition.

You can likewise take solution or over-the-counter NSAIDs (non-steroidal anti-inflammatory medications such as Vioxx, Celebrex, and Bextra), which diminish irritation, however, it can have perilous symptoms. While these medications are successful COX-2 inhibitors, the hazardous symptoms from delayed continuous use, (gastro-intestinal discharge and kidney and liver disappointment) make them both perilous and dubious. One has to peruse the writing created by the organizations producing these medications to realize how hazardous they are. Indeed, in the United States in the year 2000, additional individuals passed on from the difficulties of NSAIDs, then kicked the bucket from AIDS! Further, Vioxx was pulled back from the commercial center since it caused heart assaults.

Inflammation is 'one of the trouble makers.' You have to get it leveled out, however, don't hop from the 'skillet into the fire' by treating your condition with a 'badder person.' Eat right, practice normally, have your blood work done once per year, and tune in to your primary care physician's recommendation. May I recommend you locate a characteristic nourishment supplement to treat your aggravation, instead of simply going after the pill bottle?

How Inflammation triggers Diabetes–And Anti-Inflammatory tips to live by

Inflammation is rising as a key factor hidden in the advancement of type 2 diabetes, and it's one that numerous individuals have not known about. A typical and totally regular body reaction, irritation is a procedure by which your white platelets and body synthetic concoctions shield you from microscopic organisms, infections and disease.

You can recognize intense inflammation in your body by redness, warmth, swelling and agony at the site of damage. These are signs that your body is effectively battling a disease.

Be that as it may, under numerous conditions–regularly because of way of life factors or an over-responsive insusceptible framework–inflammation can end up perpetual, prompting a second rate condition of decay in your body. For this situation, aggravation causes no ostensibly side effects despite the fact that it might harm your system, which is the reason it's otherwise called 'quiet' inflammation.

Constant 'quiet' inflammation doesn't just involv in endless infections like coronary illness, malignant growth, Alzheimer's malady and rheumatoid joint inflammation, yet it also contributes to type 2 diabetes.

Inflammation has all the earmarks of being complicatedly connected to the improvement of type 2 diabetes. White platelets called macrophages trigger irritation as a component of your safe reaction. Macrophages additionally discharge cell-flagging synthetic concoctions called cytokines, which cause cells to move toward becoming insulin safe, a condition wherein your body has lost the capacity to use insulin fittingly, and type 2 diabetes frequently pursues.

In individuals who are fat, exploration demonstrates that macrophages move into fat tissue where they discharge cytokines and meddle with the cells' capacity to utilize insulin properly. This is an imaginable motivation behind why individuals who are overweight or corpulent are at an expanded danger of creating type 2 diabetes.

Truth be told, it's broadly realized that obesity adds to a condition of second rate 'silent' inflammation just as insulin opposition. Notwithstanding, stoutness isn't the main provocative express that can trigger insulin obstruction.

Other provocative ailments like rheumatoid joint pain, hepatitis C and fiery lung ailments are connected to an expanded danger of diabetes, which recommends that not exclusively type 2 diabetes may be an incendiary ailment too, however irritation may likewise be at fault for why heftiness triggers insulin opposition and diabetes.

Basically, the area of the inflammation or incendiary cytokines in your body will direct what wellbeing condition or indications create. For example, inflammation in your cerebrum may prompt Alzheimer's, or aggravation in your joints can prompt joint inflammation, and far reaching fundamental inflammation can prompt malignant growth and fibromyalgia..

Separate research has demonstrated that a protein called Fox01 invigorates macrophages and the creation of cytokines called interleukin-1 beta (IL-1B), leads to insulin resistance. Insulin commonly represses Fox01, which implies that when your phones are never again touchy to insulin, Fox01 can trigger irritation when unchecked.

It's an unpredictable cycle where an excessive amount of insulin is a marker for aggravation. This is the reason a fasting insulin blood test, ordinarily used to screen for diabetes, can be a marker for irritation; higher insulin levels regularly means you have higher aggravation levels.

Obviously, corpulence is one factor that is related with the quiet aggravation in your body. It's conceivable, and very normal, to have unending inflammation regardless of whether you're not overweight or large, and this is regular because of the way of how life factors work.

Your Diet and your Lifestyle Habits can increase Inflammation, too

Numerous variables can animate constant inflammation in your body, including:

1. Overweight and stoutness

2. Unhealthy eating routine

3. Poorly controlled diabetes

4. Lack of activity

5. Gum sickness

6. Smoking

7. Stress

8. Long-term contaminations

You will see numerous things on this rundown–unfortunate eating routine, absence of activity, gum illness–additionally increments your type 2 diabetes hazard, so in the event that you need to maintain a strategic distance from diabetes, it's critical to find a way to lessen the inflammation in your body.

This incorporates:

• Avoiding expert incendiary nourishments. The accompanying diets may add to foundational inflammation: trans fats (found in mostly hydrogenated vegetable oil), seared nourishments, sugar, bread and other refined carbs, soft drink, liquor and polyunsaturated vegetable oils

• Eating a lot of calming nourishments. Nourishments that help lessen inflammation incorporate crisp leafy foods, and wild-got fish (for the omega-3 fats)

• Exercising

• Quitting smoking

• Reducing worry in your life

• Consider certain calming herbs and flavors like turmeric, ginger and boswellia.

It's critical to downplay endless inflammation in your body to decrease your danger of type 2 diabetes as well as other ceaseless ailments.

How would you know whether you have endless inflammation?

The C-Reactive Protein (CRP) test is the most widely recognized test used to distinguish inflammation; it quantifies a protein in your body that increments during foundational inflammation. In one examination, ladies with raised CRP levels were observed to be about multiple times bound to create diabetes than those with lower levels, and even subsequent to modifying for other hazard factors, the hazard was still more than multiple times as high.

In any case, regardless of whether you realize you have raised CRP levels or not, it's a smart thought to make the strides above to decrease inflammation in your body. We all are affected by inflammation to changing degrees, and the best choice to keep the ceaseless, diabetes-connected sort away is to lead a solid way of life as portrayed previously.

The Inflammation-Diabetes Connection

Inflammation is the body's response to disease or damage. Exemplary indications of inflammation are redness, swelling and torment. Living in Minnesota, the model I consider is a mosquito nibble, where you feel almost no agony however you get the inflammation redness, swelling and tingling. That is a conspicuous incendiary response that is transitory.

Ever had a sinus disease? In the event that you go to the specialist you will be determined to have sinusitis. Any therapeutic determination that finishes with 'itis' signifies inflammation. So sinusitis essentially implies inflammation of the sinuses.

What does aggravation have to do with diabetes?

Diabetes and numerous perpetual medical issues are a state of inflammation, yet the unnerving part is that the inflammation is covered up. This concealed aggravation can begin its path before you realize you have diabetes. You feel no agony until it has caused intricacies that occasionally are not reversible.

Inflammation prompts insulin opposition, which means your body needs to deliver more insulin to keep blood sugars typical. At the point where your body can never again keep up, blood sugars begin to run higher than typical and all the more regularly. In the long run you may feel side effects, however many don't feel anything unique until blood sugars are in the 300s...which ismultiple times the ordinary level.

What causes Inflammation in our body?

There are several things that can cause the shrouded inflammation. Our condition, stress, dormancy, nourishment hypersensitivities or sensitivities, as well as other wellbeing conditions. The purpose behind this article...is our eating routine. Our quick paced current world methods we are presented to project unsafe synthetic concoctions. We have more pressure, we sit a lot at a work area or before a screen, and we eat unreasonably many handled nourishments.

How might you reduce your level of Inflammation?

Begin de-preparing your eating routine. That implies eat less bundled diets and more entire natural products, vegetables and entire grains. It implies less eating out and more cooking at home. Sounds straightforward, yet it's definitely not. Changing the manner in which we eat requires some serious energy, arranging and adapting better approaches for cooking and attempting new sustenance.

Where do I start?

Consider these three changes in your eating routine to begin calm eating:

1. De-processing your eating regimen.

Consider what you can do to settle on your suppers and nibble decisions, not so much prepared, but rather more new sustenance. For instance, and when you are eating canned soups, at that point begin making your very own in bigger groups and stock little in holders for fast suppers. In the event that you purchase treats, begin making custom made ones. Set a standard for how frequently seven days you can eat out and begin preparing more suppers at home. These are only a couple of recommendations to kick you off.

2. Eat progressively anti-inflammatory nourishments.

Your best source is fish such as salmon, or fish of different nourishments high in omega-3 like flax dinner. Other anti-inflammatory nourishments incorporate entire grains, crisp leafy foods and nuts.

3. Eat more fiber

Once more, entire grains, natural products, veggies and nuts are your best decisions. Rather than cold oat, pasta or moment rice, attempt some less handled grains like steel cut oats, grain, or dark colored rice. Remember to drink more water as you increment fiber.

It is proper to say that you are suffering from Chronic Inflammation?

In the event that you're eating a purported current eating routine, at that point you presumably have incessant inflammation. Nourishments like sugar, refined flours, soda pops and trans fats are generally reasons for inflammation. These nourishments are generally late augmentations to individuals' weight control plans. The human body isn't adjusted to handling these new kinds of diets, so it does not endure them greatly.

Perpetual Inflammation Symptoms

The issue is that there are frequently no undeniable indications of constant inflammation, or what signs there are we put down to some other causative factor.

That doesn't mean unending inflammation is absent in the body. An ever-increasing number of studies are demonstrating that it is one of the reasons for various infections, including coronary illness, pancreatitis, diabetes, fibromyalgia, malignancy, metabolic disorder and incessant weakness disorder. The ceaseless aggravation in the body stresses it, permitting a dependable balance for different issues.

Heftiness is additionally a noteworthy concern and adds to numerous medical issues. The cutting edge diet isn't just causing unending aggravation, it's adding crawls to our waistline. Those additional pounds cause additional inconvenience.

The Modern Diet is killing us

The new diets we've added to our eating regimen are causing issues. A portion of these professional incendiary sustenance incorporate sugar, soft drink, liquor and bread made with refined flours.

Likewise, except if you've been living under the famous shake, you've caught wind of the issues with trans fats, which are found in many nibble sustenance, fricasseed nourishments, wafers, confections, prepared products, treats, vegetable shortening, a few margarines, plate of mixed greens dressings and numerous other handled nourishments. These are found in numerous sustenance we purchase in the market, or devour at cafés, and trans fats are known to increment foundational irritation.

There are additionally synthetic substances in numerous nourishments that we truly have no clue what long haul impact they will have on our wellbeing. Too many arranged nourishments are, to a greater extent, a compound mixture than a healthy sustenance.

So if these sustenance are demolishing our wellbeing, what can be done?

Attempt an Anti-inflammation Diet

Clearly, the basic response to the issue is to change our eating routine. For some individuals, in any case, that basic answer isn't anything but difficult to actualize. It requires a move in intuition, in what nourishments we purchase and how we plan them, and what sustenance we eat when eating out.

Perusing marks is significant. In the event that you've never tried to look at the names on sustenance, there's no time like the present to begin doing it! Search for fixings known to be issues, particularly trans fats.

Abstain from eating huge amounts of handled nourishments. Rather, settle on entire nourishments, as near their characteristic state as could be expected under the circumstances. Entire nourishments are for your wellbeing diet!

Improving your Diet

It might all appear to be overpowering to make such a great deal of changes to your eating routine. And when it does, consider making child strides. Make changes in your eating regimen a little at a time, slowly improving it nibble by nibble.

Inflammation and Disease

There is a procedure in the body that is presently accepted by therapeutic specialists to be engaged with all realized sickness forms from coronary illness to malignant growth to Alzheimer's ailment–inflammation. The majority of you will have previously encountered inflammation.

Have you at any point got a chip in your finger? It got red and swollen, it might have drained a little and it was surely hot and excruciating; all the great indications of aggravation. Presently, irritation is really an ordinary reaction to damage this way and it serves us well. It eliminates microscopic organisms, parasites and infections that attempt to attack us, and this inflammation keeps us solid. This kind of inflammation, more often than not, shows a 100 overlap increment in insusceptible framework markers, for example, white platelets and cytokines like IL-6, TNF alpha, or C receptive protein (CRP).

Anyway there is another, darker fiery reaction that occurs in the body–what Dr Barry Sears calls 'Quiet Inflammation'. This sort of inflammation doesn't inspire the torment, swelling, redness and warmth related with exemplary inflammation and may just show a 4-5 crease increment in invulnerable framework markers–so it can be regularly difficult to distinguish.

It can take years to create and gradually harms DNA and prompts sickness. Sadly, present day drugs aren't truly adept at treating this kind of quiet inflammation. It is the consequence of a poor way of life decisions and the changing ways of life and sustenance that vastly improves this strategy rather than utilizing and depending on anti-inflammatory drugs.

The reasons for quiet aggravation are multi factorial:

- Over sustenance

- Excess liquor

- Poor diet

- Inactivity

- Pollution

- Poor rest

- Stress/misery

- Drug use

One of the essential wellsprings of quiet inflammation in the body is the overabundance of muscle to fat ratio. Fat isn't only an unattractive idle substance that sits on your stomach cushions or overhangs. It doesn't simply fill in as a supply of vitality to be called upon when required for vitality. Fat is a metabolic tissue that can make the way of things to occur in your body. Fat cells become invaded with large amounts of safe cells that discharge fiery synthetic substances which upset the take-up of sugar and copying of fat in liver cells by adding to insulin obstruction. This is the beginning of type 2 diabetes and narrowing corridors. Fat cells discharge synthetic concoctions that coagulation your blood, increment your pulse and convert idle pressure hormones into dynamic pressure hormones then add to conditions such as hypertension, stroke, cardiovascular ailment and PCOS.

(Bring home point - lose muscle to fat ratio)

Here is a short inflammation poll;

1. It is proper to say that you are overweight?

2. It is proper to say that you are taking cholesterol prescription?

3. It is proper to say that you are taking circulatory strain prescriptions?

4. Do you wake feeling sleepy every day?

5. Do you get sugar desires?

6. Do you experience the ill effects of weakness?

7. Do you have weak nails?

If you addressed yes to at least three inquiries, you are likely experiencing silent inflammation. In the accompanying blog entries, I'm going to disk inflammation as the course for heart assaults (not cholesterol), inflammation and circulatory strain, inflammation, malignant growth, inflammation and diabetes. I'll examine how to diminish inflammation through great nourishment.

Inflammation and coronary illness

This may be somewhat out there for some of you, particularly as we have been mentally programmed to feeling that soaked fat and cholesterol squares courses and causes heart assaults. In any case, what analysts are discovering is that inflammation is maybe the real player here, not cholesterol.

Earlier, I referenced the incendiary reaction gets activated whenever there is harm to the body. Tragically the body is under consistent low level oxidative harm all the time from free radicals. These free radicals are terrible minimal insecure particles that fly around taking electrons from cells, and for the most part, are causing ruin. The body's guard to these free radicals are cell reinforcements; cancer prevention agents that can securely give their electrons to the free radicals and render them safe. The fundamental wellspring of cancer prevention agents in our body are shaped from the nourishment we eat, sustenance that contain amino acids and supplements such as nutrient A, nutrient C, nutrient E, zinc, selenium and numerous different mixes like alpha lipoic corrosive, green tea concentrate and carotenes.

The exemplary coronary illness hypothesis looks similar to this:

• Too much cholesterol in the eating routine makes cholesterol be stored in the conduits like the coronary corridors.

• Cholesterol kept in the coronary corridors causes narrowing or blocked courses and a heart assault.

An epic way to deal with coronary illness including inflammation resembles this:

• A terrible eating routine ailing in cell reinforcements prompts poor assurance from free radicals and oxidative harm.

• As cholesterol voyages, veins move all through the vascular epithelial cells.

• Cholesterol is assaulted by free radicals and ends up harming 'oxidized cholesterol'.

• Oxidized cholesterol isn't perceived by the invulnerable system which mounts a provocative response where resistant cells called macrophages go along and eat the oxidized cholesterol.

• The macrophage that has eaten the harmed cholesterol turns into a froth cell which is presently caught inside the epithelial cells that line the dividers of the corridors.

• As these froth cells develop, they cause narrowing of the corridor and can prompt decreased blood stream to the heart muscle.

• This leads to a heart assault.

So cholesterol is the honest observer of the oxidative harm brought about by an eating routine lacking cell reinforcements.

The Mediterranean eating routine

The Mediterranean eating regimen is commonly viewed as the local eating routine of the occupants of Crete from between 1945 to 1970. It comprises of the accompanying diets:

• An abundance of plant nourishment (natural products, vegetables, heartbeats, beans and lentils, entire grains, nuts and seeds)

• Fresh natural product as the run of the mill day by day dessert

• Olive oil as the guideline wellspring of fat

• Saturated fat under 8% of all out calories

• Moderate dairy items, especially cheddar and yogurt

• Moderate fish, sheep and poultry

• Low red meat

- Less than 4 eggs every week

- Moderate wine utilization 1-2 glasses every day

- Less than 2000 calories every day

This eating regimen might be moderate to low in immersed fat, yet it is high in omega-3 fats, fiber and cancer prevention agents that help avoid inflammation.

Inflammation and hypertension

Silent aggravation adds to coronary illness as well as to hypertension or what is once in a while alluded to as hypertension. Presently, hypertension is an extraordinary illness as there aren't any perceptible manifestations in the beginning periods, so it's a smart thought to get your circulatory strain checked and do everything you can to keep it in the 'typical' zone.

A considerable amount of people have gone to the GP and had their circulatory strain estimated. They may have been informed that their circulatory strain is 120 more than 80 or 135 more than 90, however what do these numbers really mean?

At the point when your heart pulsates, it powers blood out and into the supply routes, which creates the principal number in a BP perusing. This number ought to be 120mmHg, which is viewed as typical, any higher than 140mmHg would be viewed as terrible, yet on the other hand, if that number is too low it can be awful. In any case if the courses were not solid or did not deliver some obstruction against the weight of the blood being siphoned out by the heart, the supply routes would tear open. This obstruction created by the conduits is the second number in a BP perusing. This number ought to be 80mmHg, which is viewed as typical. Any higher that 90mmHg would be viewed as awful, and alternately, if that number is too low it can be awful.

From logical research we can make estimations about your future dependent on your circulatory strain, as should be obvious. The higher your pulse the shorter your future.

- BP of 130/90 = 67 ½ years

- BP of 140/95 = 62 ½ years

• BP of 150/100 = 55 years

The corridors are not static cylinders where the blood streams, they can contract and enlarge contingent upon various factors, for example, stress, smoking and healthful status. In the event that a cylinder through which a liquid is moving river, the weight in that cylinder increments, when it broadens. The weight in the cylinder diminishes much like what occurs in supply routes.

A significant number of people would have heard that in the event that you are overweight, or eat an excess of salt, you will have higher circulatory strains, and that to decrease your pulse you have to lessen salt in the eating routine–genuine, however this isn't the main component at work here. Inflammation additionally assumes a major job in hypertension.

To comprehend this we have to get familiar with a tad about vascular science (I can see your focus going out the window, however hold on for me). The veins are fixed with endothelial cells that produce a large group of synthetic compounds that can tighten or enlarge your courses. One of the real vasodilators created by endothelial cells is nitric oxide.

Nitric oxide advises the veins to unwind and broaden, which will lessen the pulse. What we cannot deny is that C-Responsive Protein (CRP), that provocative cytokine that I referenced before, can diminish the generation of endothelial nitric oxide and increment fiery nitric oxide, prompting vasoconstriction and expanded pulse. Irritation fundamentally eats up nitric oxide. We realize that oxidative harm and free radicals decreases nitric oxide, and that hypertensive patients have diminished cancer prevention agents, for example, glutathione, superoxide dismutase, nutrient E, nutrient C, nutrient A, copper and polyunsaturated fats.

So there you have it; irritation causes expanded circulatory strain.

One thing that has appeared to decrease in the circulatory strain is something many refer to as the DASH (Dietary Approaches to Stop Hypertension) diet. The DASH diet is basically a low salt, low carb diet that is higher in protein and fundamental fats.

- Meat poultry and sleek fish 2-4 servings every day

- Vegetables 6-8 servings every day

- Fruits 4 servings every day

- Dried beans, seeds and nuts 1-2 servings per day

- Low fat dairy items 1-2 servings per day

- Cereals, grains and pasta 1-2 servings per day

- Fats and oils 4-5 servings per day (predominantly unsaturated fats like olive oil, fish oil, anyway some immersed fat is passable)

- Fibre–50g per day (blend of solvent and insoluble fiber–may need to utilize a fiber supplement)

Again, this eating regimen is lower in incendiary nourishments and higher in cell reinforcements much like the Mediterranean eating routine (in actuality there are numerous likenesses).

Inflammation and malignant growth

A developing number of malignancy specialists are arriving at the resolution that malignant growth is fundamentally a provocative malady, and that the more drawn out there is with inflammation present in a tissue or an organ, the higher the danger of related carcinogenesis.

Epidemiological investigations gauge that almost 15 percent of overall malignant growths are related with microbial contamination; this may incorporate cervical malignant growth and the HPV1 infection, gut malignant growth and provocative inside sickness because of bacterial dysbiosis and stomach disease auxiliary to H. pylori contamination. These irresistible specialists are related with a fiery reaction in the body.

One way the resistant framework manages these trespassers is to discharge free radicals that slaughter the attacking infections and microbes. These free radicals can harm the DNA of sound cells. These cells either fix themselves or bite the dust. In the event that countless cells in a zone passes on auxiliary to contamination, there is an incendiary intervened reaction that may prompt tumor development.

Numerous different malignant growths might be the consequence of long haul endless disturbance and inflammation, for example, in smoking and lung disease or compound harmfulness (xenoestrogens) and bosom malignancy. By and by there is DNA harm, inflammation cell demise and tumor development.

In the long run these tumors are equipped for discharging provocative synthetic concoctions that can keep up their development by starting the development of fresh recruits vessels that feed tumor development.

I'm not going to display a 'hostile to disease' diet, yet I will recommend that sugar could be a contributing reason to malignant growths. Malignant growth adores sugar is an explanation that appears to get united around. Malignant growth cells seem to utilize a mix of bunches of sugar and explicit proteins to disregard cell directions to cease to exist and continue developing. Furthermore, we realize that individuals who expend more omega-3 fats, cell reinforcements and fiber, experience the ill effects of malignancy. So by eating a eating routine that is anti-inflammatory such as a eating regimen wealthy in sleek fish, products of the soil may shield you from malignant growth.

Inflammation and diabetes

Inflammation may be a reason for type 2 diabetes. This sort of diabetes is commonly viewed as the consequences of being overweight and from eating an excessive amount of sugar, which makes the cells impervious with the impacts of insulin.

In any case, what may really be the reason is...irritation!

I've talked about how being overweight causes the arrival of an entire heap of incendiary synthetics that add to what is called 'silent inflammation'. Indeed, investigations on mice demonstrate that irritation incited by safe cells called macrophages (similar cells that become froth cells and lead to blocked courses, and that are moved in fat cells) prompts insulin obstruction and type 2 diabetes.

This exploration was done with mice that were hereditarily built that do not have a particular quality present in the insulin-creating cells of the pancreas. These qualities are delicate to the chronic reaction brought about by macrophages, and when these mice did not have the quality that didn't create diabetes, notwithstanding when nourished an incredibly high-fat eating routine.

This exploration was done with mice and applying it to people should be taken mindfully. There is a decent contention to diminish inflammation to ensure the pancreas.

Other anti-inflammatory nourishments that can be valuable in shielding yourself from 'quiet aggravation' include:

• Oily fish wealthy in omega-3 fats

• Ginger

• Garlic

• Turmeric

• Quercitin found in onions, broccoli, tea, wine and grapes.

Inflammation and Anti-Aging

Inflammation is, to a limited extent, a well-working insusceptible framework which invigorates a mind boggling arrangement of concoction and cell exercises performed by the body in light of damage or anomalous incitement brought about by a physical, substance or organic operator. We have all known about irritation, felt its uncomfortability and managed it in our standard ways. We don't know that free radicals inside our body are the offender of inflammation and factors into our constant life that triggers these free radicals to disturb cell work.

This article will help clarify that day by day inflammation supported over one's lifetime is the shrouded reason for maturing and sickness. It will look at the reasons for inflammation and will offer chances, through eating regimen and supplementation, to control these strange cell exercises, giving a sound age the board way of life.

Maturing is inescapable, however how one ages is a decision. A few people appear to age well, looking more youthful than their genuine birth date; others seem, by all accounts, to be ten years more seasoned than their sequential age. Our hereditary cosmetics decides how we age, however there are different factors . Therapeutic intercession has broadened life expectancy. While the normal life expectancy in 1900 was roughly 46 to 48 years; today, people can hope to live a ways into their eighties. However, how one lives these years and how well constant disease is kept under control, is profoundly subject to the maturing factors.

The 'free extreme hypothesis of maturing' looks at the components that effect our qualities and gives an establishment to how we age. In straightforward terms, the hypothesis clarifies how changes happen and how we can anticipate and defeat maturing issues that outcome from damage, disease or DNA harm. The message is that free radicals inside the body are the fundamental driver of inflammation, which brings about illness. Control free extreme harm through dietary decisions and supplementation of cell reinforcements, and you can control the harm to DNA.

Free radicals are exceptionally charged iotas that are missing one electron and makes them shaky. They enter our body through daylight, less than stellar eating routine, utilization of liquor, tobacco, airborne synthetics; even pressure and take an electron so as to increase concoction security. Most loved targets are unsaturated fats; cell layers which are wealthy in phospholipids; DNA and proteins. When focused methodical cell procedures are supplanted by the articulate disarray of electrons, that swap inevitably upsets the cell work. Free radicals are viewed as the essential offenders in maturing because they produce arbitrary radical change and deviation from a well-requested typical cell digestion. As a result, free radicals produce aggravation and day by day irritation, supported over a lifetime, is the reason for maturing and sickness. Certain indications of irritation incorporate swelling, heat, torment in joints and redness.

As we age, our guards decrease and our tissues gather the finished results of oxidative harm. We see our skin is wrinkling or maybe we are collecting 'age spots'. Within our body, oxidative pressure harms key particles fundamental to our DNA, causing malignant growth, diabetes, coronary illness, poor course and other age-related infections.

DNA is especially touchy to oxidative pressure. As electrons are stolen, they leave 'pits' in the individual strands of DNA. Free radicals cause strands of DNA to split and erode. The subsequent scratches and strand breaks influence both from working cells and undeveloped cells. Undifferentiated cell harm is incredibly pulverizing since these cells are antecedents for a huge number of various types of cells found in the body. Since the significant job of foundational microorganisms is proliferation, harmed immature microorganisms influence future ages of every single working cell. Malignancy is one malady that relies upon DNA harm. A recognizable case of this is the numerous types of skin malignancy.

Inflammation is a noteworthy guarded instrument of the body's resistant framework. When a remote body is distinguished, the invulnerable framework reacts with inflammation, which is portrayed by redness, swelling and torment at the site of contamination. Very similar things that trigger free radicals can cause irritation. Daylight, brown haze, airborne synthetic substances, horrible eating routine, liquor, medications, smoking and stress are the main reasons for inflammation.

Intense inflammation happens because of damage or disease. For the most part, inside a 24 to 48 hour time frame, this stage settle itself and recuperation procedure starts. Cell trash is expelled from the site of damage and sound substitution tissue develops. As we age, our cell reinforcement protections decrease and the oxidative harm causes perpetual chronic conditions. This sort of inflammation is increasingly drawn out. Free radicals, serious pressure and natural operators don't react to safe assault. There is no recuperation procedure and serious torment and tissue harm happens. Beating these conditions and switching maturing relies upon effective DNA fixs. Our inquiry is how we help nature along with a fixed procedure for DNA and invert maturing? One path is through eating in a routine and with supplementation. Another way is how you lead your life. The two methodologies are decisions.

A suitable eating routine, supplementation and positive way of life are basics to forestalling inflammation, killing free radicals and advancing solid age the board. Among our decisions, there are corrosive and soluble based nourishments. Diet should comprise of 80% soluble diets and 20%

acidic nourishments. A rainbow determination of six servings of foods grown from the ground, natural at whatever point conceivable, can guarantee this immeasurably significant corrosive/basic parity lessening aggravation through furnishing the body with a huge number of cell reinforcements. Carrots, pumpkin, peppers, tomatoes, mangos and papaya are generally orange and 'red coded' and secure our qualities. Asparagus, broccoli, bok choy, onions and mustard greens are 'green coded' and help improve cell supplements and detoxify our body. Blackberries, fruits, beets are purple and blue and diminish inflammation. Grain, mushrooms, tofu and wild rice are tan and lessen insulin opposition and parity hormones. Herbs and flavors such asgarlic, turmeric, cinnamon, curry, ginger and cayenne help to kill free radicals.

By and large, meats, grains, nuts and sugar are acidic and advance unfortunate free radicals. Meats ought to be unfenced, implying that they are free of hormones and anti-microbials. One ought to have an eating routine of ranch raised salmon, tilapia, flop and sardines. Keep away from swordfish, which is known to be high in mercury. Grain, quinoa, dark colored rice and wild rice are superb selections of grains. Nuts and seeds are essential to a balanced eating routine. Dull verdant greens, vegetables, and red, yellow, orange and green vegetables must be overwhelmed by every feast in order to adjust the important acidic nourishments which offer us the genuinely necessary protein nutrients and minerals our body needs. We can further diminish irritation with elevated amounts of antacid water admission, green tea and maintain a strategic distance from sugar, vinegar, salt and corn syrup. More or less; stress lean natural protein and join vegetable sources, eat specifically, stay away from sugary desserts, nitrates, nitrites, smoked meats and trans-fats. Watch segment sizes, don't eat on the run and bite your sustenance. You ought to have five servings of leafy foods; ideally green and orange red shading choice. Drink a lot of fluids between dinners; no soft drink, eat suppers at ordinary occasions; don't eat late and dodge handled diets. Diminish dairy utilization. We are the main species that expends another species milk!

Numerous anti-inflammatory enhancements are cancer prevention agents and help our body control free extreme harm. Superb multi nutrient/mineral complex is basic to a sound way of life. Folic acids, B nutrients, nutrients D, C, and E, boswella, glucosamine-chondroitin, curcumin, molecularly refined omega-3 and 6 from virus water fish trimethylglycine, CoQ enzyme 10, r-lipoic acid, and resveratrol are for the most part supplements that will hinder illness movement and diminish inflammation.

Nutrients A, C, and E bring down the danger of coronary illness. They decrease inflammation and ensure against initiated oxidative harm. Those with diabetes can see improvement in 'insulin activity'. Green tea secures against estrogenic bosom disease. Nutrient D3 counteracts colon malignant growth and matured garlic averts harm to DNA and furthermore diminishes inflammation. For the most part, by expanding detoxification, we free our groups of free radicals.

The utilization of the compound CoQ10 has critical outcomes in controlling maturing. This enhancement counteracts oxidative harm to the cerebrum, upgrades expedient recuperation and cardiovascular capacity from heart assaults and forestalls thyroid issue. Alpha-Lipoic corrosive improves sugar digestion, improves mind vitality and solid skeletal execution and 'splashes' up free radicals inside the body.

Diet, supplementation and learning are the key fixings to age the board. In any case, way of life changes total the whole picture in advancing life expectancy. Research demonstrates that pressure starts significant changes in cell structure that lead to maturing ailments, especially those including inflammation and invulnerable capacity.

Work towards disposing of pressure and you draw out life expectancy. Day by day exercise, supplication and reflection are additionally positive powers to fuse into one's life. Figure out how to be careful, build up an association with your God and think 'comprehensively'. Lessen liquor utilization, help your stomach related procedure with probiotics, create legitimate disposal and reduction acidic nourishments. There is no enchantment projectile, yet a longing for health turns into a way of life that comes bearing significant presents for an existence of feeling better and looking great. Genuine magnificence originates from inside. There are no alternate routes!

CHAPTER SEVEN

FOODS TO AVOID

This anti-inflammation diet is a program used to anticipate and lessen the dangers of heart sicknesses. A supper ought to be made out of 40% sugars, in addition to 30% protein and another 30% for sound fats. Suppers must be prepared on time. It is ideal to get ready at any rate and abstain from eating a similar sustenance in excess of five times each week. They contain up to multiple times more nutrients and minerals. Additionally, picking natural nourishments decreases your introduction to pesticides.

In following the counter inflammation diet, there is no restriction to the measure of nourishment that you can devour. Here are the instances of nourishment that you can eat:

1. Steamed vegetables are profoundly prescribed to improve the use and the accessibility of the sustenance supplements. This will enable the body to begin fixing itself. Then again, eating crude vegetables ought to be done negligibly aside from when having plates of mixed greens. In any event, one kind of green vegetable should to be incorporated into the eating regimen consistently.

2. Any vegetables can be eaten, however tomatoes and potatoes ought to be kept away from until further notice. It is ideal to pick and eat vegetables that are low in glycemic sugar, from about 3-6%. A few vegetables with 3% glycemic starch are asparagus, broccoli, celery, cucumber, lettuce, spinach, parsley and watercress. Vegetables with 6% glycemic starch incorporate string beans, eggplant, leeks, red pepper, pumpkin, turnip and zucchini. Carrots, squash, green peas and artichokes have 15%, while yam has 20% glycemic starch.

3. It is fitting to eat one to two bits of organic products with the exception of citrus. It's ideal to have the organic product heated.

It might be not very simple to design nourishment for an enemy of irritation diet, yet positive changes in the body will happen and results can be perceptible in about a month and a half.

Decreasing Inflammation by choosing the right Natural Food

Nourishment is the most ideal approach to improve any wellbeing condition, yet sustenance can aggravate it more. Decades back sustenance was no issue. We ate the sustenance that was accessible and it didn't influence our wellbeing since it was all normal back then. The assortment of nourishment and preparing has expanded and this is the place the issues begin. With regards to inflammation and joint inflammation related torment, picking an inappropriate sustenance can exacerbate it and disturb that circumstance considerably more.

Studies have shown that over 40% of those individuals around the planet are experiencing and identifying fiery ailments due to the form of diets that they consume. What is more, a significant degree of these do not consider the typical calming nourishments they need to integrate in their weight management programs. At the stage when a particular disease increases its horrible mind there's a reason for this particular; there has been a cause point in order for it to happen. Why are a couple of individuals becoming powerless to pollution in the transferable disease than other people, often only a normal virus? Have you ever seen people scarcely ever get whatever as where others possess some bug that's coasting about?

Immune System

Our body has a safe system which is in charge of dismissing any sickness that goes along, or it can open the entryway and give it access. The resistant framework comprises of various capacities, for example, a body detoxification framework, the provocative and anti-inflammatory system. In the event that lopsidedness happens in any of those systems by not getting the correct supplements, this will expand the danger of any disease including any sort of malignant growth. The urgent point is if sustenance disappointment happens, any sort of sickness is practically unavoidable.

Diets that reason irritation

These are a portion of the provocative nourishments, an absolute necessity to maintain a strategic distance from:

• Refined sugar

• Any sort of handled sugar

• Artificial sugars

• Any high clycemic starches

• Refined grains

• Vegetable oils

• Excessive liquor

• Processed financially raised meats

• Avoid generally oils and trans fats

Regular eating plans do not work for everyone. You will find in each event some people react badly to some decent and powerful eating regimes. Tune into your own body, it is going to let you know.

Battling Inflammation with Food

If you encounter the ill effects of joint inflammation and joint torment, or constant infections like diabetes and coronary illness, you should realize that inflammation in the body can aggravate manifestations

Diet can help battle irritation in your body. Actually, eating an eating regimen rich in anti-inflammatory nourishments can improve any irregular hormone characteristics and can offer numerous different advantages like:

• Improved vitality

• Reduction in joint and muscle torment

• Less joint swelling

• Improved portability

• Improved processing with less swelling and gas

- Bowel normality

- Clearer thinking

- Reduction in migraines

- Better quality rest

- More stable dispositions

- An improvement of fasting glucose levels and lower lipid levels

Diets that fight Inflammation (And those that don't)

Most importantly, and when you need to lessen irritation in your body, you should maintain a strategic distance from:

- Refined sugars and grains like white flour, white rice and table sugar

- Junk sustenance and cheap food. They regularly contain awful fats (trans fats) that exacerbate irritation

- Foods that reason sensitivities like wheat, dairy and eggs can build irritation

• Saturated fats. Changing to low fat dairy items and lean meat may help

• Processed meats like lunch meats, franks and frankfurters. They contain nitrites and sulphites that can advance aggravation

• Too much omega-6 fats–safflower, corn and sunflower oils

To bring down irritation in your body, do the following:

• Drink close to 6 to 8 cups of water each day

• Balance the omega-6 in your eating routine with omega-3. Use margarine and additional virgin olive oil

• Eat an assortment of splendidly hued vegetables and natural product every day

• Eat chicken, profound water fish, vegetables and beans more regularly than red meat

• Eat seeds, nuts and their margarines. Ground flax, pumpkin seeds, just as sesame and sunflower seeds, are incredible decisions

• Avoid singed sustenance more often than not

• Eat an assortment of grains other than wheat–quinoa, buckwheat, cereal, darker rice, millet

• Avoid sugar, particularly table sugar. Extremely modest quantities of maple syrup, grain syrup, nectar or stevia can be utilized when required

Continuously utilize the 90/10 standard when picking diets to battle irritation: 90% of the time, adhere to the above rules; the other 10% of the time, cut yourself a little room to breath. What's more, tune in to your body. And when your body has torment or any of different side effects recorded above, observe what you have eaten and lessen that sustenance in your eating regimen to check whether it has any kind of effect.

Mitigating Foods to add to your Diet

I don't get inflammation's meaning? It's anything but a contamination, despite the fact that disease can cause inflammation. All things considered aggravation is the body's own safeguard endeavor to evacuate unsafe upgrades, for example, aggravations, harmed cells and so forth. This is when inflammation is attempting its recuperating procedure.

Inflammation is the principal sign when something destructive or bothering is influencing portions of our body. Each one's body has an insusceptible framework and aggravation is a piece of that. Inflammation is a limited physical condition that outcomes as a response to damage or disease, making portions of the body become swollen, blushed, agonizing and hot. Inside irritation can occur because of the eating of handled nourishments, fats and sugars.

Large amounts of irritation can cause various wellbeing intricacies like joint inflammation, joint torment and harm to veins. To battle this, it is significant you eat sustenance that are calming. Such diets are promptly accessible to add to your eating routine to control irritation. Here are a portion of the diets and recommendations to help and keep hurtful inflammation under control:

Whole Grains

With regards to entire grains it is better you expend your grains as entire grains. Research has demonstrated that entire grains contain a high measure of fiber which decreases the fiery marker in blood known as C-responsive protein.

Dark Leafy Greens

Dull verdant vegetables such as spinach and kale have high centralizations of nutrient E and minerals like calcium and iron. Studies demonstrate that nutrient E helps in shielding your body from provocative atoms known as cytokines. Moreover, dim verdant greens have a high measure of malady battling phytochemicals.

Fatty Fish

Sleek fish, for example, salmon and fish are diets that are mitigating as they contain high measures of omega-3 unsaturated fats. The unsaturated fats are known to help joint inflammation, so ensure you get a lot of omega-3. Another significant truth about omega-3 is you should get it in your diet in light of the fact that the body can't make it inside its framework.

Soy

Soybeans contain isoflavones mixes which help the negative impacts of aggravation on joints. In any case, it is great you evade vigorously handled soy items as they may contain added substances and additives. Rather, incorporate soy milk and soy beans into your normal eating regimen.

Nuts

Nuts like almonds and pecans are wealthy in nutrient E, calcium and fiber. All nuts are brimming with cell reinforcements, which can help the body in fixing the harms brought about by inflammation.

Berries

Berries are low in fat and calories, however they're wealthy in cell reinforcements. Their anti-inflammatory anthocyanins compound in them has numerous great characteristics. This keeps you from creating joint inflammation.

Green Tea

Green tea also has anti-inflammatory flavonoids; this diminishes the beginning of irritation and limits the danger of specific malignant growths. It shouldn't be thought little of for some since it has other medical advantages. It can reactivate skin cells causing skin to seem more splendid. Drink it consistently and utilize some nectar as a sugar rather than sugar.

Low Fat Dairy

Low fat dairy such as yogurt, contains probiotics which can forestall inflammation. Moreover, dairy sustenance that are calming like skim milk with high calcium and nutrient D, are significant for everybody since separated from having anti-inflammatory properties. They also reinforce your bones.

Ginger and Garlic

Ginger and garlic are sustenance that are mitigating. Both are known to lower body inflammation, control glucose levels and help your body in battling certain diseases. Selenium and sulfur in garlic is a fundamental compound for a solid safe framework. It is one of the top enemies of maturing sustenance you can eat.

Turmeric and Sweet Potato

Turmeric has common mitigating mixes called curcumin, which is known to mood killer NF-kappa B protein that triggers the procedure of aggravation. Then again, sweet potato is a decent wellspring of fiber, nutrient B6, nutrient C, complex sugars and better carotene.

These fixings help to mend inflammation in your body. These are some of numerous diet that are anti-inflammatory which can help you in diminishing joint torment and joint pain brought about by aggravation. Add them to your eating routine. Notwithstanding, decrease diet that are high in fats particularly trans fats and sugar as they can prod inflammation, joint torment, joint inflammation and harm veins among other related chronic conditions.

Rolling out a couple of improvements will improve numerous things and can make them feel more lively and invigorated than you have in quite a while, and will keep on doing as such as long as you remain with the progressions you made. At the point when things have improved they return to a similar old path as in the past. Try not to attack your very own wellbeing; stick with what you are doing, the progressions you made, that made you feel much improved. Try not to return to the old ways what you've done previously.

How Can Anti-Inflammatory Diet protect you from disease?

Inflammation is something worth being thankful for. It is the regular way your body reacts to dangers. We have all observed irritation at work when we have agony and redness at damage. We state it looks excited, and it actually is, on the grounds that damage actuates the fiery reaction.

When is inflammation an issue?

At the point when inflammation goes on for significant lots of time, we call it a constant and it can cause issues. Some basic reasons for unending inflammation incorporate sensitivities, immune system ailment, periodontal ailment, joint inflammation and different illnesses that actuate the safe system after some time. Indeed, even heftiness is provocative, on the grounds that fat cells emit synthetic substances considered cytokines that trigger aggravation.

For what reason is it an issue?

Endless inflammation makes harm the endothelial covering of corridors, which can prompt atherosclerosis and coronary illness. There is proof that it adds to type 2 diabetes, Alzheimer's sickness and a developing number of other constant maladies that are basic in present day, western social orders.

What are the side effects?

The side effects of inflammation fluctuate with what is causing it. You may even have no manifestations by any means, as on account of heftiness. Here are a few instances of explicit sickness related side effects:

• Arthritis, rheumatoid joint pain (joint torment, firmness, swelling)

• Crohn's malady or ulcerative colitis (stomach torment and cramping, fever, loose bowels)

• Psoriasis or skin inflammation (redness)

• Allergies (respiratory manifestations, hives)

Increasingly unobtrusive, early markers of issues could incorporate cerebral pains, muscles hurts, exhaustion, muscle firmness, queasiness, regurgitating, the runs or blockage, gas, stomach uneasiness and even passionate issues including wretchedness. These could be identified with diet sensitivities and bigotries. The most well-known sustenance bigotries incorporate dairy (lactose), wheat (gluten), yeast, soy, corn, eggs and even some counterfeit sugars.

How might you know whether you have constant inflammation in the event that you don't have indications or a conclusion?

You can see whether you have inflammation by having your C-receptive protein levels tried. The high affectability C-receptive protein, is the favored marker of endless, poor quality inflammation.

What can you do if you have large amounts of C-responsive protein?

In the event that your C-receptive protein levels are high, you will initially need to converse with your primary care physician to see whether there is a hidden contamination, sensitivity, immune system issue or other contributing malady. If not, your overabundance weight could be the reason and weight reduction is your best line of safeguard. And when you are a smoker, that could be adding to the issue.

How do nourishments impact inflammation?

Inflammation can be affected by the diet you eat. Research has demonstrated that specific nourishments trigger inflammation and others smother it.

A portion of the nourishments that are star incendiary include:

• Animal fats (corn-encouraged hamburger, dull meat and skin of poultry, pork, duck)

• Hydrogenated fats (trans fat)

• Fried nourishments (browned in saturated, hydrogenated or polyunsaturated fats)

• Sweets (sugar, treats, treats, cakes, dessert, doughnuts, sweet drinks)

• Refined grains (white bread, pasta, and white rice)

• Processed diet (chips, saltines, fries, cold cuts, sausage, canned meats)

• Dairy items (particularly full fat milk, cheddar, harsh cream, cream cheddar, cream)

• Some individuals may need to maintain a strategic distance from the nightshades (potatoes, tomatoes, eggplant, peppers)

Here are the best mitigating diet:

• Fatty fish likesalmon, sardines, herring, trout and fish (with omega-3 unsaturated fats)

• Grass sustained hamburger contain some omega-3 fats (not at all like corn-nourished meat, generally soaked fats)

• Nuts and seeds (pecans, flaxseed, almonds)

• Monounsaturated fats (olive oil, canola oil, avocados), by supplanting polyunsaturated fats

• Turmeric (some portion of most curry dishes)

• Ginger, utilized in Asian cooking (additionally helps control sickness)

• Whole grains (with the exception of wheat, grain and rye and when you are gluten bigoted)

Nourishments that have high cell reinforcement levels will decrease inflammation, perhaps by diminishing the harm that invigorates inflammation. Cell reinforcements are productive in splendidly and obscurely shaded foods grown from the ground.

The absolute best wellsprings of cell reinforcements include:

• Berries: blueberries, raspberries, blackberries, cranberries, strawberries, fruits

• Beans: red beans, kidney beans, pinto and dark beans

• Herbs: oregano, basil, sage, marjoram, thyme, dill, garlic, dry mustard

• Spices: cinnamon, cloves, cumin, turmeric, ginger

• Nuts: walnuts, pecans, pistachios

• Green tea is wealthy in the two cancer prevention agents and mitigating mixes

• Coffee, cocoa (or dim chocolate) and red wine (yet caffeine and liquor are provocative)

• Exotic organic products: acai, gogi, pomegranate, papaya, pineapple

Eating a greater amount of these mitigating and high cancer prevention agent diets can help quiet incessant irritation and decrease your hazard for endless infections. Discover approaches to make these nourishments a piece of your regular eating regimen, and you won't just shield your body from malady, yet you may locate that a portion of your throbbing painfulness will improve.

The Anti-Inflammatory Diet for Arthritis Relief

Sustenance and joint inflammation have an association with one another and that is the reason changing your eating regimen is one of the primary recommendations a specialist can give an individual with aggravation in their joints. There are nourishments that can lessen the aggravation and there are those that may intensify the irritation. An individual with joint pain ought to pursue the anti-inflammatory diet in the event that the person needs to get treated. To begin a mitigating diet, one should know which diet the individual in question is going to wipe out in one's eating routine and which nourishments will be included.

What is the diet that you ought to maintain a strategic distance from and take out in your eating routine?

With regards to joint inflammation, it is constantly exhorted that the individual influenced ought to take out counterfeit diets like low quality nourishments, those diet that have been handled and diet with included fake flavorings and colorings. An individual with joint pain ought to maintain a strategic distance from meats that have large amounts of fats and nourishments that are high in sugar.

The reasons why these sorts of nourishments ought to be maintained a strategic distance from by individuals with joint pain is that the immersed fats and trans fats found in these diets can exacerbate one's condition. The person in question ought to keep away from potatoes, eggplants and tomatoes on the grounds as these are a piece of the nightshade group of plant that contains solanine, which can incite the torment. Cutting these sorts of vegetables in individuals with joint pain have not been demonstrated at this point to be viable, however the individuals who pursued this sort of eating routine regularly show enhancements with their condition and discover alleviation from torment.

What are the diet to be included your eating regimen and when you have joint pain?

In the event that you definitely know which sorts of nourishments you ought to kill in your mitigating diet, you should now realize diet to add to your eating routine:

1. Solid fats and oils: Fish oils are high in omega-3 unsaturated fats and are basic to our wellbeing. This will help diminish the inflammation and keep it from returning. You will get these fats in certain seeds like flaxseed, pumpkin seeds and sunflower seeds and furthermore in Brazil nuts, almonds and cashew nuts.

2. Foods grown from the ground: You ought to eat more products of the soil when you have joint inflammation. These foods have a great deal of mineral, nutrients and cancer prevention agents that are advantageous for your joint pain and to different conditions.

3. Protein: Eating more proteins like fishes, different seafood and poultry meats will help individuals with joint inflammation.

4. Beverages: You should require more fluids to keep your joints greased up. Drink more water, natural product juices, tea, vegetable juice with low sodium and non-fat milk.

Treating yourself for joint pain isn't troublesome, and when you know the sort of eating diet that is proper for your condition, and in the event that you realize the diets to maintain a strategic distance from,

CHAPTER EIGHT

Dieting Protocol – Meal Plan And Recipes

In this healthy 1200-calorie supper plan, the standards of a mitigating diet meet up for seven days of scrumptious, healthy dinners and tidbits, in addition to feast prep tips to set you up for a fruitful week ahead, which would take you through a 30-Day venture.

The buzz encompassing inflammation and its association with constant ailments and wellbeing conditions like joint inflammation, diabetes, heftiness, gut issues and coronary illness may leave you pondering, "What is a calming diet?" and "Should I tail it?"

An anti-inflammatory diet is tied in with eating a greater amount of the diet that help to squash inflammation in the body, while constraining the nourishments that will increment inflammation, subsequently combatting provocative conditions. The eating regimen accentuates heaps of bright products of the soil, high-fiber vegetables and entire grains, sound fats (like those found in salmon, nuts and olive oil) and cancer prevention agent rich herbs, flavors and tea, while constraining prepared diets made with undesirable trans fats, refined starches (like white flour and included sugar) and an excessive amount of sodium. In this sound 1200-calorie supper plan, we pull together the standards of mitigating eating to convey seven days of heavenly, healthy dinners and bites, in addition to feast prep tips to set you up for a fruitful week ahead.

Since inflammation can be brought about by a lot of different factors other than nourishment, similar to low movement levels, stress and absence of rest, joining the solid way of life propensities into your every day schedule can help avert inflammation. To get the most anti-inflammatory advantages, pair this solid dinner plan with standard physical movement (go for 2 1/2 hours of moderate action every week), stress-diminishing practices (like yoga, reflection or whatever works best for you), and a decent night's rest each night (at any rate seven hours out of every night). Regardless of whether you're attempting to effectively diminish inflammation or are just searching for a healthy eating plan, this 7-day anti-inflammatory feast plan can help.

Step by step instructions to meal-prep your week of meals:

A little feast prep toward the start of the week will set you up for good dieting achievement.

1. Prep the Vegan superfood buddha bowls to have for lunch on Days 2, 3, 4 and 5. Refrigerate bowls and dressing independently for as long as four days. Hold back to add avocado until prepared to eat to avoid sautéing.

2. Make the Turmeric-ginger Tahini dip to have with snacks consistently.

Day 1

Anti-inflammatory bonus: foods high in omega-3 unsaturated fats such as salmon, sardines and tuna fish, have been appeared to diminish irritation levels and intend to incorporate two 3-ounce servings of fish high in omega-3 unsaturated fats every week.

Breakfast (287 calories)

- 1 serving Blueberry-banana overnight oats

- 1 cup green tea

A.M. Bite (31 calories)

- ½ cup blackberries

Lunch (325 calories)

- 1 serving Green salad with edamame and beets

P.M. Bite (117 calories)

- 2 Tbsp. Turmeric-ginger Tahini dip

- 1 medium carrot, cut into sticks

Supper (442 calories)

- 1 serving Walnut-Rosemary Crusted Salmon

• 1 serving Roasted squash and apples with dried cherries and pepitas

Every day totals: 1,202 calories, 57 g protein, 131 g starch, 30 g fiber, 54 g fat, 1,520 mg sodium

Day 2

Anti-inflammatory bonus: vitamin C, a cancer prevention agent, has mitigating benefits since it helps decline hurtful free extreme cells that may trigger inflammation. Studies demonstrate that individuals who have eats less carbs high in nutrient C have lower levels of the provocative marker C-receptive protein just as lower danger of incendiary infection, similar to gout and coronary illness. The present Raspberry-kefir power smoothie gives 45 percent of the suggested every day esteem for Vitamin C!

Breakfast (249 calories)

• 1 serving Raspberry-kefir power smoothie

A.M. Bite (28 calories)

• 1/3 cup blueberries

Lunch (381 calories)

• 1 serving Vegan superfood buddha bowl

P.M. Bite (9 calories)

• ½ cup cut cucumber prepared with a squeeze every one of salt and pepper.

Supper (393 calories)

• 1 serving Indian-spiced cauliflower and Chickpea salad

• 5 ounces unsalted canned tuna fish, in water (depleted)

Top plate of mixed greens with fish.

Night Snack (156 calories)

- 1 ounce dim chocolate

Day by day totals: 1,215 calories, 70 g protein, 143 g starch, 35 g fiber, 47 g fat, 1,054 mg sodium

Day 3

Anti-inflammatory Bonus: Anthocyanins are ground-breaking cancer prevention agent mixes found in dull blue, red and purple foods grown from the ground, just as red wine. Research demonstrates that anthocyanins assume a job in diminishing inflammation markers, which can decrease danger of malignancy and coronary illness. Keep solidified berries available for a calming lift to your morning smoothies or oats so you can get the advantages notwithstanding when they are not in season.

Breakfast (263 calories)

- 1 cup low-fat plain Greek yogurt

- 1 ½ Tbsp. slashed pecans

- ¼ cup blueberries

- 1 cup green tea

Top yogurt with pecans and blueberries.

A.M. Tidbit (42 calories)

- 2/3 cup raspberries

Lunch (381 calories)

- 1 serving Vegan superfood buddha bowl

P.M. Tidbit (117 calories)

- 2 Tbsp. Turmeric-ginger Tahini dip

- 1 medium carrot, cut into sticks

Supper (409 calories)

- 1 serving Superfood chopped salad with salmon and creamy garlic dressing

Day by day totals: 1,212 calories 77 g protein, 97 g starch, 28 g fiber, 63 g fat, 813 mg sodium

Day 4

Anti-inflammatory bonus: Eating dull chocolate and cocoa with some restraint may diminish irritation markers and improve heart wellbeing. Cocoa is rich in the flavonol quercetin, which is an amazing cancer prevention agent that secures our cells and the reason dim chocolate is a significant part in the calming diet. Consolidate one 1-ounce square multi day of the darkest chocolate you can discover to boost benefits.

Breakfast (222 calories)

- 1 serving Cocoa-chia pudding with raspberries

A.M. Bite (109 calories)

- ½ cup low-fat plain Greek yogurt

- ¼ cup blueberries

Lunch (381 calories)

• 1 serving Vegan superfood buddha bowl

P.M. Bite (9 calories)

• ½ cup cut cucumber

• Pinch of salt

• Pinch of pepper

Supper (472 calories)

• 1 serving Stuffed sweet potato with hummus dressing

Every day totals: 1,191 calories, 56 g protein, 168 g sugar, 49 g fiber, 39 g fat, 1,100 mg sodium

Day 5

Anti-inflammatory bonus: Probiotics, similar to those found in kimchi, yogurt, kefir and fermented tea, help bolster a solid gut. Research demonstrates a sound gut improves our invulnerable frameworks, keeps up a solid weight and lessens aggravation. Likewise, make sure to incorporate prebiotics, which are unpalatable plant strands found in sustenance like garlic, onions and entire grains that help give fuel to great microbes to upgrade our gut wellbeing.

Breakfast (249 calories)

* 1 serving Raspberry-kefir power smoothie

A.M. Bite (2 calories)

* 1 cup green tea

Lunch (381 calories)

* 1 serving Vegan superfood buddha bowl

P.M. Bite (58 calories)

* 1 Tbsp. Turmeric-ginger Tahini dip
* 3/4 cup cut cucumber

Supper (414 calories)

• 1 serving Korean steak, kimchi and cauliflower rice bowl

Night Snack (120 calories)

• 5 ounces red wine

Every day totals: 1,224 calories, 57 g protein, 112 g sugar, 28 g fiber, 53 g fat, 1,067 mg sodium

Day 6

Anti-inflammatory bonus: More than 20 percent of U.S. grown-ups are influenced by some type of joint pain, which is a provocative malady of the joints, which is regularly treated with a blend of an anti-inflammatory diet and doctor prescribed medicine. The best anti-inflammatory diet routine for joint inflammation incorporates a lot of magnesium. Inquire about demonstrates that it diminishes irritation and keeps up joint ligament. Most people don't get enough magnesium, so make sure to incorporate a lot of vegetables, nuts, entire grains, dim green verdant vegetables and seeds to guarantee satisfactory admission.

Breakfast (249 calories)

• 1 serving Raspberry-kefir power smoothie

A.M. Tidbit (157 calories)

• 12 pecan parts

Lunch (325 calories)

• 1 serving Green salad with edamame and beets

P.M. Tidbit (78 calories)

• 1/2 ounce dim chocolate

Supper (401 calories)

• 1 serving Hummus-crusted chicken

• 1 serving Blistered broccoli with garlic and chiles

Feast Prep Tip: Cook and hold additional chicken to have with lunch tomorrow. You'll require 2 cups hacked cooked chicken.

Day by day totals: 1,209 calories, 73 g protein, 94 g starch, 28 g fiber, 63 g fat, 1,245 mg sodium

Day 7

Anti-inflammatory bonus: An eating routine high in fiber will have a lower glycemic record, which is a proportion of how nourishments sway our blood sugars. Fiber is processed gradually, which keeps us full and improves glucose control. A special reward—eating sustenance lower on the glycemic list—may help lessen levels of C-responsive protein, which is a marker for inflammation. This solid mitigating plan gives in any event 28 grams of fiber consistently.

Breakfast (292 calories)

• 1 serving Cocoa-chia pudding with raspberries

- 1 Turmeric latte

A.M. Tidbit (42 calories)

- 1/2 cup blueberries

Lunch (350 calories)

- 1 serving Avocado egg salad sandwiches

P.M. Tidbit (116 calories)

- 15 unsalted almonds

Supper (448 calories)

- 1 serving One-pot garlicky shrimp and spinach
- 1 cup cooked quinoa

Day by day totals: 1,209 calories, 62 g protein, 128 g sugar, 32 g fiber, 55 g fat, 1,362 mg sodium

Added Anti-Inflammatory diet strategies

• Drink unsweetened tea and coffee. Avoid sodas and other drinks that contain sugar

• Should you drink alcohol, then select red wine and beverage in moderation. A chemical found in red wine, resveratrol, has anti inflammatory properties

• Satisfy your teeth by selecting dark chocolate

Foods you should avoid on an Anti-Inflammatory Diet

Similarly as significant as eating more foods that battle inflammation is eating less nourishments that may cause irritation. Pursue these rules to free your eating regimen of sustenance that may build aggravation in your body.

• Avoid profoundly handled nourishments made with white flour and sugar, similar to white bread and bundled snacks and prepared merchandise

• Reduce your admission of immersed fat by eating less full-fat dairy, including spread, cream and high-fat cheddar. Greasy meats contain high measures of soaked fat, as do items made with palm oil and coconut oil

• Cut back on creature proteins, including red meat, cheddar and yogurt. Concentrate your protein admission on omega-3-rich fish and plant sources

CONCLUSION

An anti-inflammatory diet was not created in light of weight reduction, yet all things considered, eating a eating routine high in some low-calorie, supplement thick sustenance, similar to natural products, vegetables and beans, and low in handled nourishments and included sugars, will prompt weight reduction. One thing to note is that albeit high-fat sustenance like avocados and nuts are gainful, they are additionally high in calories. Be aware of your segments when picking these diets.

Considering these certainties, it's critical to realize that a calming diet has not been demonstrated to battle inflammation related ailments, however the nourishments and dietary patterns the eating regimen elevates have been appeared to have heap medical advantages.

In general, an anti-inflammatory diet is a sound method for eating that is in accordance with eating nourishment gauges. This eating routine advances what we've known up and down: a sound eating routine incorporates organic products, vegetables, entire grains and solid fats. Constraining prepared, browned, refined, sugary diets is a smart thought for a more beneficial eating routine, as a lot of those kinds of nourishments may prompt the advancement of perpetual ailments. Following this eating routine should expand your nutrient, mineral and fiber admission and will probably make you feel more beneficial and perhaps help you shed pounds.

I kindly ask you to do me a favour and leave a good review for eBook on Amazon. So, please, just go to your account on Amazon…

Thank you and good luck!